The Affordable Care Act as a National Experiment

Harry P. Selker • June S. Wasser
Editors

The Affordable Care Act as a National Experiment

Health Policy Innovations and Lessons

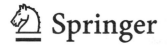 Springer

Editors
Harry P. Selker, MD, MSPH
Dean
Tufts Clinical and Translational Science
   Institute
Tufts University

Executive Director
Institute for Clinical Research
   and Health Policy Studies
Tufts Medical Center
Boston, MA, USA
hselker@tuftsmedicalcenter.org

June S. Wasser, MS
Instructor in Medicine
Tufts University School of Medicine
Boston, MA, USA
June.Wasser@tufts.edu

ISBN 978-1-4614-8350-2   ISBN 978-1-4614-8351-9 (eBook)
DOI 10.1007/978-1-4614-8351-9
Springer New York Heidelberg Dordrecht London

Library of Congress Control Number: 2013945223

Printed on acid-free paper

Springer is part of Springer Science+Business Media (www.springer.com)

*This volume is dedicated to the memory of
Senator Ted Kennedy, a long-time champion
of universal healthcare access and
healthcare research who was an inspiration
to many who care about these issues and
who contributed more than any other
individual to the possibility of this book.*

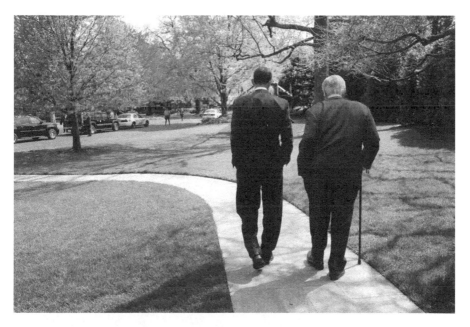

President Barack Obama and Senator. Ted Kennedy walking down the South Lawn sidewalk at the White House. Color image. April 21, 2009. Official White House photo by Pete Souza

Foreword

It was a long way from my former desk in the chamber of the US Senate to my operating room where we transplanted hearts back in Nashville. But I've built my career on the understanding that policy has consequences for behavior.

From conceptualization and development of health policy to implementation and execution is a path that allows for continued shaping and reshaping. To maximize constructive consequences, and minimize the unintended negative, a useful framework for looking at new policy is to view it as research.

This book takes on two challenging tasks: (1) describing the far-reaching Patient Protection and Affordable Care Act (ACA) and (2) making the case that innovations such as the ACA are research that is fundamental to our nation achieving the healthcare system it deserves and needs.

The description of the messy development and initial implementation of the ACA, its novel approaches to improve our nation's access to, and quality of, care, and such unexpected events as the Supreme Court decision of June 2012 make this book a rewarding read. Moreover, as a policy maker who worked hard to support more value-driven health reform and health service research and as a clinical investigator at Vanderbilt University School of Medicine who focused on "translational research" that directly impacts patient care, I fully agree with the construct that new policies are really experiments.

One thing that we all know is that our very stressed medical sector will not fix itself. It will require innovation and experimentation—and we as a nation must understand and support that. Like laboratory research, health policy research requires careful observation. It is difficult but holds great promise.

From the very beginning, it was clear that the ACA would not—and could not— solve all of the challenges in the healthcare landscape with broad strokes. Access is more than coverage. The drivers of healthcare costs are profoundly varied and complex. The policy would need to be explored and examined over time, continually refined by both public and private sector stakeholders.

The ACA presents an enormous opportunity to carefully observe healthcare policy and measure our progress. This collection of studies looks at the value for patients, discusses the goals of information technology in healthcare, and discusses metrics by which we can evaluate our progress.

As we look ahead to a more modern American healthcare system, we must keep sight of both the staggering need for reform and the continued complexity of the process. Healthcare in the future will require more input and engagement than ever before—from patients and physicians and policy makers. The Affordable Care Act was not the solution to a broken healthcare system, but the beginning of a new era of work.

Ultimately, the ACA is only one (very large) piece of a puzzle that we as a nation must solve to better understand and optimize our healthcare system. As the Preface states, "The ACA may be the largest healthcare experiment in our history, but it is far from being the last." I am confident that this book will inform and motivate many others to participate in and support this critical work—our nation and our health depend on it.

William H. Frist, MD
Former Majority Leader, US Senate

Preface

Now seen in overview, the construction and passage of the Patient Protection and Affordable Care Act (ACA) in 2009–2010, including its many innovations, may seem quite logical and orderly. However, the process of its creation was anything but orderly, and many of the hurdles it had to survive and/or accommodate defied logic. Its becoming law was a fight—or, more aptly described, a riot. There were so many different constituencies looking to advance their points of view and interests that the scene was less a pro vs. con two-sided war than a civil war among many factions— some in alliances and some freelancing. Now as the nation experiences the implementation of the ACA, although there remains contention and some uncertainty, as established law, it is the framework for our health system for the coming years.

Innumerable individuals and organizations, some well known and some anonymous, were involved in, and contributed to, the ultimate legislation and its landmark passage, including the authors of the chapters in this book. Some of the authors were deeply involved in creating the preconditions that enabled the ACA, such as the Massachusetts universal healthcare experiment. Some helped write the ACA bill and helped with its ultimate passage. Some are involved in its implementation. And some have been involved in all of these efforts. The ACA's creation will discernibly improve individuals' and our nation's medical and economic health. Thus, we owe thanks to those who have made these contributions and written the chapters that follow, as well as for their contributing these perspectives and stories about the ACA.

All policy innovations can be seen as experiments. Accordingly, as explained in the initial chapter, we see the ACA not only as landmark legislation but also as the largest health policy experiment our nation has ever undertaken. We emphasize this aspect in this book because it highlights the importance of learning from this innovation and the importance of healthcare research to improving—indeed, perhaps saving—our nation's healthcare system.

In the first section, the chapters by Kavita Patel and by Shawn Bishop, who both were deeply involved in the writing of the ACA bill, tell of the creation of the ACA. Much of the approach was based substantially on the results of a preceding experiment, healthcare reform in Massachusetts, echoing Justice Brandeis's comments in 1932, "It is one of the happy incidents of the federal system, that a single courageous state may, if its citizens choose, serve as a laboratory; and try novel social and economic experiments without risk to the rest of the country" [1]. The results are detailed in the chapter by Massachusetts Secretary of Health and Human Services, JudyAnn Bigby, as well as in the chapters by major participants in that experiment, John McDonough, James Roosevelt, Jr., and Brian Rosman. A newer state-based experiment in expanding healthcare access, ongoing in Vermont, enabled by the ACA, is described in the chapter by Anya Rader Wallack, who is leading that effort.

This book's accounts of the development of the ACA illustrate that, unlike experiments in the lab or the clinic, healthcare policy experiments have protean real-world challenges—including initial and continuing political opposition in many forms. The stories in this volume emphasize an unalterable feature of translational research as one looks to translate biomedical research from the bench to the bedside, to clinical practice, to general public benefit, and to policy; the "laboratory" becomes increasingly less controlled by the experimenter and more subject to random or even intentional interference. One of the most remarkable examples of this was the state attorneys' general suit to have the law overturned by the US Supreme Court, reviewed in Chapter 14. Although that did not end the experiment as had been wished by some, it did have an effect on the results of the experiment. Chapter 15 reports on the impact of the Supreme Court's decision on states' implementation of Medicaid expansion, still unfolding. Other hurdles to the execution of the ACA experiment have been more predictable but not less important, such as the need to create a national health information technology infrastructure, as laid out in Chapter 8. Another challenge, in common with any major policy innovation, has been the need for public engagement. The challenge of this is illustrated in the juxtaposition of Chapter 11 by Bruce Landon and Stuart Altman that portrays the ACA's value proposition for our nation and Chapter 12 by Ceci Connolly that depicts how that value was—or was not—successfully communicated. June Wasser's commentary in Chapter 10 lays out how we might hope this will go better in the future.

Looking to the future, John McDonough, in Chapter 16, outlines the key next experiments in healthcare reform, and the commentaries by James Roosevelt and by Brian Rosman remind us that the ACA is a major step but only one on a longer path of understanding and optimizing our healthcare system. The reader will recognize many things that remain to fulfill the ACA's objectives and to learn how best to deliver healthcare to our nation. The ACA may be the largest healthcare experiment in our history, but it is far from being the last. We hope this volume will help inform future innovations in the crucial but still distant objective of a more perfect healthcare system.

Boston, MA, USA   Harry P. Selker, MD, MSPH
                                                                              June S. Wasser, MS

Reference

1. Greve MS. Laboratories of democracy: anatomy of a metaphor. [May 2001]. Available from: http://www.federalismproject.org

Acknowledgments

The authors thank Muriel Powers and Tiffany Bagby for coordination of and expert preparation of the book manuscript, Amy west for editorial assistance, Randi Triant for final editorial coordination and oversight, and the Springer staff for facilitating the publishing of this book.

This project was supported by the National Center for Research Resources Grant Number UL1 RR025752 and the National Center for Advancing Translational Sciences, National Institutes of Health, Grant Number UL1 TR000073. The content is solely the responsibility of the authors and does not necessarily represent the official views of the NIH.

Contents

Contributors

Stuart Altman, PhD The Heller School for Social Policy and Management, Brandeis University, Waltham, MA, USA

JudyAnn Bigby, MD Formerly Health and Human Services, State of Massachusetts, Boston, MA, USA

Shawn Bishop, MPP Marwood Group, Washington, DC, USA

Craig Brammer HealthBridge, Cincinnati, OH, USA

Terence Burke Denterlein, Boston, MA, USA

Ceci Connolly, BA Former National Health Correspondent, Washington Post, Washington, DC, USA

Paul Jean Denterlein, Boston, MA, USA

Bruce E. Landon, MD, MBA, MSC Department of Health Care Policy, Harvard Medical School, Boston, MA, USA

John McDonough, DPH, MPA Center for Public Health Leadership, Harvard School of Public Health, Boston, MA, USA

Kavita Patel, MD, MS Engelberg Center for Health Care Reform, Brookings Institution, Washington, DC, USA

James Roosevelt, Jr., JD Tufts Health Plan, Watertown, MA, USA

Brian Rosman, JD Health Care For All, Boston, MA, USA

Harry P. Selker, MD, MSPH Tufts Clinical and Translational Science Institute, Tufts University, Boston, MA, USA

Institute for Clinical Research and Health Policy Studies, Tufts Medical Center, Boston, MA, USA

Anya Rader Wallack, PhD Green Mountain Care Board, Montpelier, VT, USA

June S. Wasser, MS Tufts University School of Medicine, Boston, MA, USA

Mallory West Engelberg Center for Health Care Reform, The Brookings Institution, Washington, DC, USA

Chapter 1
Introduction: The Affordable Care Act as a National Experiment

Harry P. Selker

Over the last several years, the US public has witnessed a political fight about government policy on a scale and intensity not seen in decades. Perhaps surprisingly, this no-holds-barred political fight has been about whether, how, and to what extent the nation should expand healthcare insurance coverage to 30-plus million currently uninsured citizens. The strategies and tactics have included both the ordinary and extraordinary. The responsible Congressional committees' staff (including authors of chapters in this book) drafted legislation in the usual way—although aware that the stakes were unusually high. However the tactics used to influence legislators and the public were beyond the usual, such as the description of payment for physician time to discuss end-of-life planning with their patients as "death panels." The polarization of messages was such not seen since the Vietnam War era.

In this context, in many quarters, it might not help the debate to point out that the proposed healthcare reform was essentially an *experiment*. But it is, indeed it is the biggest healthcare experiment in our nation's history. This book is an accounting of the rocky initiation of this massive experiment and some early signals about its results.

Of all that might be said about the Patient Protection and Affordable Care Act (ACA)—one of the most important and most challenged pieces of legislation in our nation's history—why emphasize that it is an experiment? The opportunity to portray the American public as "guinea pigs" in research facility cages would do little to improve the discourse. Then why advance this concept? First, it should be appreciated by all involved that any major policy innovation is an experiment. There will be hypotheses and expectations, but until implemented and tested, we cannot be certain of the results, so we need to collect data on the impact of innovations.

H.P. Selker, M.D., M.S.P.H. (✉)
Tufts Clinical and Translational Science Institute, Tufts University, Boston, MA, USA

Institute for Clinical Research and Health Policy Studies, Tufts Medical Center,
Boston, MA, USA
e-mail: hselker@tuftsmedicalcenter.org

H.P. Selker and J.S. Wasser (eds.), *The Affordable Care Act as a National Experiment:*
Health Policy Innovations and Lessons, DOI 10.1007/978-1-4614-8351-9_1,
© Springer Science+Business Media New York 2014

Additionally, for the public, a better understanding and appreciation of the importance of healthcare experiments and research, including at the policy level, could help generate public support, which would be a good influence. Also, for those who work in this area, it is worth taking a step back from the fray and seeing that while Martin Luther King, Jr., promised that the arc of history bends towards justice [1], it is important to recognize that real innovations are required to create that bend towards universal access to healthcare. Thus, this book's frame for policy innovations is intended to make explicit that the nation needs to learn from the challenges of doing such experiments.

The public is fascinated by, and conceptually supportive of, medical and healthcare research, as documented by Research!America [2]. When asked, 71 % of Americans believe that research is a solution to rising healthcare costs, and 87 % are willing to share their health information through electronic health records if that would help health officials better understand causes of disease and disability. Moreover, majorities of Americans believe that the national commitment to health research should be yet higher and that comparative effectiveness research will improve healthcare. However, if not asked, or if guided by contrary messaging, although crucial to their actual experience of medical care and new treatments, many people do not consider healthcare delivery and policy research to be part of the chain of medical research. Just as care is advanced by bench-to-bedside research that translates biological insights into effective treatments, the public needs to understand that care also is advanced by bedside-to-practice-to-public-benefit-to-policy translational research. New treatments, or even customary treatments, if not delivered effectively to individuals, have no impact on health [3]. Widespread understanding of the need for this full spectrum of research would lead to better public support, including better understanding of the process of policy innovation.

It should be understood that because policy innovations are experiments, plans and results are not easily predicted, and often in-course adjustments are needed. For example, recently the Administration delayed a year, until 2015, the ACA mandate that employers of over 50 people provide health insurance to all their workers. More time is needed to have the requisite systems in place to properly implement, monitor, and enforce the mandate. The actual impact is minor: the vast majority of 50-plus employee businesses already provide health insurance to their workers—the delay only will affect about one percent of the nation's workers. We need to understand that such adjustments are the inevitable consequence of the policy innovation process, and one such as this, practically, will not hold us back.

Not only is it important for the public to understand the benefits of healthcare research, the government itself also could better demonstrate this understanding. Although the ACA has improved the picture a bit, the balance of health research supported by our government is heavily tilted towards support for the basic and bench-to-bedside research, done by the National Institutes of Health (NIH), funded at 100 times the level of the agency that does healthcare delivery research, the Agency for Healthcare Research and Quality (AHRQ). Considering the complexity of this country's healthcare delivery system that is crucial to delivering medical care and advances, and considering the massive costs of healthcare, AHRQ and its type of research might be justified as being 100-fold *larger*, not smaller, than NIH. Or at least it could be justified as deserving to be on the same scale. Moreover, just as the Food and Drug Administration (FDA) requires that new drugs be demonstrated to be safe and effective before being allowed for widespread use, so should there be a government interest in the safety and effectiveness of healthcare delivery policies.

Those of us in health policy and healthcare research also need to better embrace this narrative. If we cannot articulate why this work is important and how it will inform and improve the nation's health, we undermine our own objectives. We must make the case that the value of this work should be widely understood as a crucial part of research across the entire spectrum of translational research—from bench-to-bedside-to-practice-to-public-benefit-to-policy. Research that fails to traverse this entire chain, that is, fails to keep a clear line of sight on the ultimate potential health benefit, will not provide ultimate benefit.

Besides attempting to make this case, this volume describes the largest such experiment, the institution of the ACA, to make clear just how challenging such an endeavor is. Its scale and cost are enormous, yet the public, government, and those in healthcare delivery and policy research all must understand and support it as critical for progress on one of our nation's unfulfilled obligations—to provide for the optimal health and function of all our residents.

Measured in billions of dollars, millions of people, and thousands of pages of legislation and supporting regulation, the ACA is arguably the most expansive and ambitious healthcare innovation—experiment—ever undertaken in this country. It seeks to extend healthcare coverage to tens of millions of US citizens and to simultaneously make the healthcare system more economically sustainable and thereby to benefit all Americans. In service of these goals, the ACA is already being evaluated by the US Department of Health and Human Services (HHS) Office of the Assistant Secretary for Planning and Evaluation (ASPE), as reflected in reports available at http://aspe.hhs.gov/health/reports/2012/ACA-Research/index.cfm:

- Affordable Care Act Expands Mental Health and Substance Use Disorder Benefits and Federal Parity Protections for 62 Million Americans
- Estimated Savings of $5,000 to Each Medicare Beneficiary from Enactment Through 2022 Under the Affordable Care Act
- Overview of the Uninsured in the United States: A Summary of the 2012 Current Population Survey Report
- 47 Million Women Will Have Guaranteed Access to Women's Preventive Services with Zero Cost-Sharing under the Affordable Care Act
- Number of Young Adults Gaining Insurance Due to the Affordable Care Act Now Tops 3 Million
- The Affordable Care Act and Asian Americans and Pacific Islanders
- The Affordable Care Act and African Americans
- The Affordable Care Act and Latinos
- Uninsured Young Adults and the Affordable Care Act
- The Affordable Care Act and Women
- The Affordable Care Act and Participation Rates in Medicaid

- Expanded Insurance Coverage For Young Adults of All Races and Ethnicities
- 105 Million Americans No Longer Face Lifetime Limits on Health Benefits
- ACA and Preventive Services Coverage Without Cost-Sharing
- The Cost of Covering Contraceptives through Health Insurance
- Medicare Beneficiary Savings and the Affordable Care Act
- At Risk: Pre-Existing Conditions Could Affect 1 in 2 Americans
- The Affordable Care Act and Children
- Comparing Health Benefits Across Markets
- Essential Health Benefits: Individual Market Coverage
- Variation and Trends in Medigap Premiums
- 2.5 Million Young Adults Gain Health Insurance Due to the Affordable Care Act
- Actuarial Value and Employer-Sponsored Insurance
- One Million Young Adults Gain Health Insurance in 2011 Because of the Affordable Care Act
- Overview of the Uninsured in the United States
- The Value of Health Insurance: Few of the Uninsured Have Adequate Resources to Pay Potential Hospital Bills

In addition, many other federal and state agencies and Congressional bodies are evaluating the impact of this experiment, as are many independent academic and research organizations. There will be many questions about the ACA healthcare policy experiment—and data on its impact will be forthcoming.

Aside from being an experiment itself, the ACA supports healthcare research. As centers for this research, it created the Center for Medicare and Medicaid Services (CMS) Innovation Center and the Patient Center Outcomes Research Institute (PCORI). The CMS Innovation Center is detailed in a later chapter in this volume, and the creation of PCORI (in which this author was involved) and the attendant controversy are described in the chapters by Kavita Patel and by Shawn Bishop about the development of the ACA legislation. Both of these research entities focus on generation and translation of best evidence and best practices into widespread use, in support of improved healthcare and the execution of the ACA, and illustrate the span of health policy research.

The CMS Innovation Center supports research, demonstration, and implementation projects that will benefit healthcare delivery and value. Under the ACA, it receives $10 billion over 10 years. Uniquely and importantly, the ACA provides for direct translation of positive results into Medicare rules by the Secretary of HHS, thereby greatly accelerating their having impact. Thus the Innovation Center is an example of research set up to maximize the impact of the ACA in helping CMS achieve "the triple aim" of improving the experience of care, improving the health of populations, and reducing per capita costs of healthcare.

In contrast, PCORI is outside of the government, governed by a Board composed of a wide range of stakeholders in healthcare. With funding of $4 billion through 2019, it is focused on comparative effectiveness research (CER) and its translation into improved patient-centered care. Its research is intended to inform patients, care providers, and the public about the comparative effectiveness of treatments and care strategies in making critical healthcare decisions, in support of the ACA's goal of effective healthcare.

By creating the CMS Innovation Center and PCORI, the ACA strengthened the role of research in improving the quality, effectiveness, and value of healthcare. By creating these two new research entities, with mechanisms linking them to implementation, the ACA is putting translational research at the center of American healthcare improvement. Along with the many improvements the ACA makes in American healthcare financing and delivery, we now have the opportunity that all translational researchers seek, to have real impact on health.

Biomedical and healthcare research are critical to our nation—especially important is translation into ultimate care and health. This work is vital, and in support of this, it is crucial that the nation appreciate the importance of research and experimentation—along the entire spectrum of translational research. We hope this volume will contribute to this understanding.

References

1. Martin Luther King, Jr. Speech, Montgomery, AL; 1963.
2. Research!America: America Speaks. Alexandria, VA; 2009.
3. McGlynn EA, et al. The quality of healthcare delivered to adults in the United States. N Engl J Med. 2003;348(26):2635–45.

Part I
Implementing Change: Objectives of the ACA

Chapter 2
Commentary on Part I: Objectives of the ACA

James Roosevelt, Jr., Terence Burke, and Paul Jean

Even before the outcome of the November 2012 presidential and congressional elections abruptly terminated the electoral challenge to the Patient Protection and Affordable Care Act (ACA), President Obama's signature policy accomplishment had already set in motion transformative changes to the nation's healthcare system that are unlikely to be reversed. Although many of its most important provisions will not go into effect until 2014, the ACA has begun the process of expanding access to care, correcting widespread abuses and inequities in the health insurance markets, improving the quality of care, enhancing preventive care, and facilitating the emergence of new healthcare delivery and payment systems.

The ACA stands as one of the most far-reaching pieces of social and economic legislation in US history. It rightfully takes its place alongside Social Security, Medicare, and Medicaid as watersheds in advancing a more equitable and just society. The ACA represents the first time the USA has enshrined access to health care as a fundamental right of *all* citizens and a dramatic federal governmental restructuring of the healthcare insurance market and delivery system.

The passage of the ACA responded to powerful economic and social pressures in American society—rising numbers of uninsured and underinsured Americans; unsustainable increases in the cost of health care, with healthcare expenses approaching 20 % of GDP; a rising tide of chronic disease that threatens to actually *reverse* gains in life expectancy; and a growing realization that the failures of its healthcare system and the health of its citizens are matters of vital US national interest, with powerful implications for economic growth. As Kavita Patel recounts in Chap. 3, "Delivering on the Promise of the Affordable Care Act" Obama administration

J. Roosevelt, Jr., J.D. (✉)
Tufts Health Plan, Watertown, MA, USA
e-mail: James_roosevelt@tufts-health.com

T. Burke • P. Jean
Denterlein, Boston, MA, USA
e-mail: tburke@denterlein.com; pjean@denterlein.com

H.P. Selker and J.S. Wasser (eds.), *The Affordable Care Act as a National Experiment:*
Health Policy Innovations and Lessons, DOI 10.1007/978-1-4614-8351-9_2,
© Springer Science+Business Media New York 2014

officials were fond of pointing out that Americans spend twice as much on health care alone as Chinese consumers spend on all personal consumption.

The following two chapters by Kavita Patel of the Brookings Institution and by Shawn Bishop of the Marwood Group, both of whom were Senate staff to the relevant committees (Health, Education, Labor and Pensions, and Finance, respectively) involved in writing the ACA, examine the goals of the ACA, what the ACA does (and does not do), and how implementation of the bill will determine its long-term impact. What seems beyond doubt is that "Obamacare" portends nothing short of revolutionary change in US health care, and the success of this law will determine the domestic policy legacy of President Obama in much the way Social Security did for President Franklin Delano Roosevelt and Medicare and Medicaid did for President Lyndon Johnson.

ACA: Systemic, Revolutionary, Innovative, and Catalytic

Systemic

In 2006, Massachusetts passed landmark health reform legislation aimed at providing universal access to health insurance coverage. Massachusetts policymakers deliberately chose to limit the scope of the law to expanding coverage (through policy tools such as an individual mandate, subsidized insurance and health insurance exchanges) and to postpone action on the complex issues of cost control, payment reform, and quality of care. Thus, Massachusetts took a sequential approach and only in 2012, after succeeding in extending health insurance to more than 98 % of its residents, did it pass major follow-on legislation addressing rising healthcare costs and healthcare delivery and payment reform.

The Obama administration, which drew much of its inspiration for the ACA from the 2006 Massachusetts health reform law, eschewed the state's gradual approach and decided to tackle the issues of access, cost, quality of care, and payment reform simultaneously. This systemic approach was premised on a recognition of the interrelatedness of these issues blended with a good deal of political realism: that the administration would need to be able to make tradeoffs between different aspects of the law to secure support from key stakeholders and that it was likely only to get one bite at the health reform apple. Despite the political deals built into the law, Patel points out that it is remarkable how consistent the bill's many provisions are and, we might add, how they fit together to advance the law's main goals.

One example of this is how the ACA addresses its primary objective of extending health insurance coverage to a large portion of the 50 million Americans without it. The ACA utilizes several interlocking policy tools to create a "continuum of coverage," which with one exception were left intact by the Supreme Court's June 2012 decision.

First, the law enacts several insurance market reforms which prohibit private insurers from engaging in a range of all too common practices that have had the effect of restricting access to health insurance. These practices included denying coverage or charging higher prices as a result of preexisting medical conditions, charging women higher premiums than men, retroactively terminating coverage for individuals who become sick, and imposing annual or lifetime caps on benefits.

Second, the Supreme Court left in place the most controversial aspect for enhancing affordability: the individual mandate. This provision was adopted to prevent people from "free riding" (not paying for insurance but still benefitting from guaranteed access to care and thus shifting costs onto other consumers) and to protect insurers and the market from the consequences of "adverse selection" where individuals acquire insurance only when they get sick.

Third, the ACA called for a significant expansion of Medicaid to cover an estimated 16 million people by 2019. This provision recognized that an individual mandate alone would not suffice when many people without health insurance are unable to afford the premiums.

Now, as laid out in Chaps. 11 and 12, the Supreme Court's decision has essentially made the Medicaid expansion optional rather than mandatory for states. At press time, 24 states are moving forward with Medicaid expansion, 21 are not moving forward, and six are debating it, according to the Kaiser Family Foundation. JudyAnn Bigby's second chapter (15) gives a report on this as of Spring 2013. Several Republican-controlled states have expressed strong opposition to it, although much of that may have reflected political grandstanding prior to the 2012 elections. The ACA contains strong incentives for states to adopt the expansion. The federal government picks up the vast majority of the tab and, as the Urban Institute estimates, states overall would realize a net fiscal *gain* of between \$40 billion to \$130 billion from 2014 to 2019. And it is precisely those states that have been most vociferously opposed that would in fact have the most to gain; Texas, for example, would see 49 % reduction in uninsured adults with incomes at or less than 133 % of the federal poverty level (FPL).

The final element of expanded access is the formation of state insurance exchanges, similar to the Commonwealth Health Connector in Massachusetts, where consumers earning between 133 % and 400 % of FPL will be able to purchase insurance assisted by a sliding scale of federal subsidies.

Health and Human Services Secretary Sebelius waived or extended the 2013 deadline to encourage states to adopt exchanges. As of this writing, 17 states have declared that they will have exchanges, seven are planning "Partnership Exchanges," a state-federal hybrid, and 27 states are defaulting to the federal government to create their exchange, according to the Kaiser Family Foundation.

Revolutionary

The ACA does not stop at expanding access to coverage and care. As Bishop points out "delivery system reform is actually the bulk of the bill… and what makes the bill truly new and revolutionary."

The ACA shuns a cost-cutting approach; there are undoubtedly costs that could be pulled out of the system through unit price reductions, but this is not where the big efficiency gains will come from. As the most innovative healthcare organizations like Geisinger Health System have recognized, organizations can "simultaneously improve quality, satisfaction and efficiency only by redesigning and reengineering the delivery of care" [1].

The law embodies several elements that are designed to improve care coordination and encourage healthcare providers to take "responsibility for the total experience of care," as Atul Gawande frames it in his provocative "Big Med" essay in *The New Yorker* [2]. Under the ACA, for example, hospitals would receive reduced payments from Medicare and Medicaid if too many patients are readmitted to the hospital within 30 days. Rather than being *rewarded*, hospitals are now assuming *risk* for patients being readmitted. This provision thus incentivizes hospitals to be more diligent in following up with discharged patients to make sure they are following the discharge care instructions and seeing their primary care physician.

Perhaps most revolutionary are the provisions in the ACA designed to move providers away from fee-for-service methodologies and toward bundled payments (for episodes of care) and global payments (for defined populations over a given period of time). While paying for results, not services, hardly seems like that groundbreaking of a concept, in medicine this marks a radical break with how physicians have been compensated from time immemorial. Both bundled and global payments encourage providers to shift their focus from volume to the value of care they deliver and to "manage their transitions of care, the different settings that patients move to in a course of treatment, in a much more efficient way" (Bishop).

Innovative

One of the more forward-looking aspects of the ACA is that it builds in mechanisms for continuous healthcare innovation. As Bishop points out, "we left a lot of things out [of the bill] … because we didn't know enough to say whether certain things were sound public policy." Rather than seek to be overly prescriptive during a period of extraordinary change in health care, the law creates mechanisms "to make reform self-sustaining." The foremost example of this is the Center for Medicare and Medicaid Innovation, which was created to develop, test, and disseminate innovative payment and care delivery models that emphasize care coordination and efficiency. The Center was capitalized "with $10 billion every 10 years to create experiments on how to evolve the healthcare system as we learn about what might work." If the center generates ideas that show considerable promise, the Secretary of Health and Human Services "gets to take those ideas national without having to go to Congress for approval" (Bishop).

The ACA does not stop at system reform. As a fundamental purpose of the law is to drive improvements in healthcare quality, it also establishes the Patient Centered Outcomes Research Institute (PCORI). The purpose of PCORI will be to conduct comparative effectiveness research to test to determine the relative clinical effectiveness of different healthcare products and procedures. It is estimated that fewer than half of all care decisions made in the USA are based on adequate scientific evidence. Understanding the clinical effectiveness of different products and procedures relative to their cost will also be vital to controlling healthcare spending and directing scarce resources toward their most impactful and effective use.

Catalytic

While the ACA marks a dramatic break from the past, it does not, as many Republican critics have charged, represent a federal takeover of the healthcare system. The ACA preserves the predominant role in the healthcare system for private providers and insurers and affords the states significant latitude over implementing many provisions of the law.

Under the ACA, the federal government assumes an expanded role in the healthcare system, but that role takes more of the form of a catalyst and partner rather than command and control. One way to think of the federal role is that of midwife to birthing a more effective healthcare system. The ACA acknowledges the central role of the market in advancing reform but plays a critical part in providing direction and facilitating that change.

The ACA creates a framework for the establishment of private accountable care organizations (ACOs) in Medicare and establishes a shared savings program under which ACOs may earn additional payments by exceeding certain cost and quality benchmarks. The law establishes several demonstration and pilot projects for supporting the market's shift away from fee-for-service payment methodologies to bundled and global payments.

Further it leverages the power of Medicare and Medicaid to drive change in healthcare delivery and improving the quality of care. As Patel discusses in her chapter, the Center for Medicare and Medicaid Innovation is bringing a new level of transparency to healthcare quality and performance measures with the implementation of so-called five-star ratings for Medicare Advantage plans. Under this system, those plans that receive scores of three stars or better based on quality metrics will receive bonus payments from Medicare. The goal is to reward plans that facilitate more coordinated and efficient care.

Implementation

In her chapter, Patel advances a strong argument that the effectiveness of federal healthcare reform will be shaped by the complicated interplay of foreseen and unforeseen events, intended and unintended consequences, that occur when designated agencies and other bodies try to implement the new law. There are of course numerous uncertainties going forward, even with the legal and political uncertainty having been definitively resolved by the Supreme Court and the voters: will the Obama administration bargain away important provisions of the ACA in budget and debt negotiations with House Republicans? If the administration traded away the most unpopular provision, the individual mandate, but kept popular aspects such as guaranteed issue and/or community pricing, would this lead to dramatic increases in health insurance premiums? Will Republicans continue to try to sabotage the ACA by attempting to de-fund its implementation? Will some states have more success with their exchanges than others? How many and which states will finally implement the Medicaid expansion? How many people will resist obtaining health insurance and decide instead to pay the "tax" for violating the individual mandate? How many employers will cease providing health insurance and pay the penalty for employees who receive subsidies through an exchange?

As we move forward with the ACA, in some ways there are more questions than answers because so much of this is new. But the experience in Massachusetts does provide some confidence that some of the adverse unintended consequences have not in fact come to fruition. As one example, there was concern that many businesses in Massachusetts would drop health insurance coverage for their employees altogether and let their employees obtain insurance through Commonwealth Connector—Massachusetts insurance exchange. However, not only has business not walked away from providing health insurance, the business-backed Massachusetts Taxpayers Association has reported that the number of small businesses offering health insurance has *increased* from 70 % to 77 %.

That is not to suggest we should be sanguine about the possibilities for unforeseen outcomes. However, one of the virtues of the ACA is that it is designed to be a flexible instrument that allows learning from and responding to experience.

Conclusion

Kavita Patel opens her discussion of the origins of the ACA 1 with the observation that the immediate impetus for the ACA was the widespread recognition that time was running out on healthcare business as usual. That reality remains every bit as relevant now as it was in 2009–2010. Despite the controversy surrounding the ACA, we can think of no healthcare executive who truly doubts that the healthcare system is in need of serious reform.

What is different is that the ACA has already begun to have a significant impact on the market. Even before the 2012 elections finally killed the hopes of ACA opponents, the ACA had set in motion transformative changes to the nation's healthcare system that are unlikely to be reversed, including the ACA's reforms that correct widespread abuses and inequities in the health insurance markets.

Most importantly, the market has already anticipated the ACA's impact in moving the system from fee-for-service to different payment models that reward quality, coordination, and efficiency of care. Providers and payers across the country are already experimenting with new payment models in their contracts, creating improved systems for delivering care and developing new evidence-based care protocols. The ACA will further facilitate these changes and help bring them to scale, but the reform train has already left the station. There are going to continue to be strong—we would even say irresistible—economic pressures to continue moving the system from volume to value.

Finally, the public has now spoken through the ballot box in recognizing ACA as the law of the land. "Obamacare" is indeed a reality, and the ACA will indeed define this president's legacy for years to come.

References

1. The Commonwealth Fund Case Study, Geisinger Health System: Achieving the Potential of System Integration Through Innovation, Leadership Measurement, and Incentives. June, 2009.
2. Gawande A. Big Med *The New Yorker*, August 13, 2012.

Chapter 3
Delivering on the Promise
of the Affordable Care Act

Kavita Patel and Mallory West

Observations are often made about the differences between a prospective law's aims, its final shape after the legislative process, and its effects in the real world. The complications of getting major legislation through Congress and signed into law are paralleled by the complicated interplay of foreseen and unforeseen events and intended and unintended consequences that occur when designated agencies and other bodies try to implement the new law. This situation can be aptly applied to the passage of the Patient Protection and Affordable Care Act (ACA). Chris Jennings, senior health policy advisor to President Bill Clinton, wrote in the *New England Journal of Medicine* that "the legacy of [the ACA] will be determined by the underlying policy and the competence with which it is implemented." [1]

Complete repeal of the Patient Protection and Affordable Care Act is highly unlikely; however, final implementation is still dependent on a number of factors. The ACA was born in the maelstrom of politics and its final implementation will certainly be influenced by the ever-changing political landscape. Republicans will look to target specific reforms for repeal, most notably the Independent Payment Advisory Board. Other provisions within the ACA have received bipartisan support and have already been piloted. However, close analysis of these demonstration projects underscores the verity that expected and actual outcomes do not always align. With political and market forces equally contributing to the capricious nature of legal implementation, how do we know when we have delivered on the promise of increased access, better quality, and lower costs? For this reason, the ability to test, evaluate, and disseminate results over regular intervals is intrinsic to successful implementation of the ACA.

K. Patel, M.D., M.S. (✉) • M. West
Engelberg Center for Health Care Reform, Brookings Institution, Washington, DC, USA
e-mail: kpatel@brookings.edu; mlwest@brookings.edu

H.P. Selker and J.S. Wasser (eds.), *The Affordable Care Act as a National Experiment: Health Policy Innovations and Lessons*, DOI 10.1007/978-1-4614-8351-9_3,
© Springer Science+Business Media New York 2014

Access Expansion

The ACA aims to increase access to health insurance by providing a continuum of affordable coverage options. Expanding access to Medicaid and creating health insurance exchanges are integral to achieving this goal. Under the original language of the ACA, Medicaid eligibility was to be expanded to all non-Medicare eligible individuals under the age of 65 with incomes up to 133 % federal poverty level (FPL). In addition, states would maintain current income eligibilities for seniors and persons with disabilities, while low-income children (those between 100 and 133 % FPL) currently covered by the Children's Health Insurance Program (CHIP) would be transitioned to Medicaid. The federal government promised to fund 100 % of costs associated with covering the newly eligible for the first three years and 90 % of the cost thereafter. The projected addition of 15–16 million lives to Medicaid by 2019 held great promise in promoting health equality for disadvantaged groups and reforming payment models to recognize those providers who sustain care to low-income individuals [2].

However, in June of 2012, the Supreme Court ruled that the Medicaid expansion was unconstitutionally coercive of the states for two reasons. First, the states were not given adequate notice to voluntarily consent to the expansion. Second, the original language stated that the secretary could withhold all existing Medicaid funds for noncompliance. While the Supreme Court decision effectively limited the federal government's ability to enforce the Medicaid expansion, it did not invalidate the language of the ACA rather, it gave states the option to refuse part or all of the new eligibility requirements. State governors now will have to decide whether to move forward with the expansion, a decision made more difficult by those states with a divided government. How will political pressure from the electorate influence the states' decisions? Will the states use this as leverage against the federal government or will the reverse be true as the states are pressured to take on the expansion? How will the adoption or rejection of the expansion coincide with the legislative cycle? The Medicaid expansion is at the mercy of the shifting political landscape.

Whether states choose to adopt the new eligibility requirements or not further highlights the importance of developing proof points at regular intervals. The Congressional Budget Office first projected that 23 million people would remain uninsured after implementation of the ACA. The Supreme Court decision changed those calculations and new estimates report a net total of 29 million uninsured Americans by 2022 [3]. Further analysis allows one to identify trends and populations most at risk. For example, legal and undocumented noncitizens constitute 22 % of the uninsured population [4]. While undocumented residents are not eligible for Medicaid regardless of income, legal residents have a 5-year waiting period before becoming eligible for Medicaid. States have the option of expanding Medicaid coverage to legal immigrant children and pregnant women within this 5-year window; however, the stipulation still leaves many uninsured. Research must address the question of the uninsured, updating final counts and highlighting those populations most at risk. These data points will help assure that we are delivering on the promise of increased access to disadvantaged groups.

The ACA also hopes to expand coverage by mandating the creation of state-based health insurance exchanges. Requiring that Americans purchase health insurance necessitates that affordable coverage options are available. To achieve the goal, the exchanges offer affordable, comprehensive coverage options to qualified individuals and small businesses. The exchanges will serve as a common marketplace that consolidates the available choices and provides consumers with transparent data on cost and quality. In addition, the exchanges will pool risk for small groups and regulate consumer cost sharing to promote efficiency and contain costs.

States have the decision to pursue a state-based exchange, a partnership exchange, or a federally-facilitated exchange. At this writing, 27 states have reported that they will not move forward with establishing a state-based health insurance exchange and will instead default to a federally-facilitated exchange. Seventeen states have declared a state-based exchange while the rest are planning for a partnership exchange. However, there is little information on how the federally-run exchanges will operate and how states will be integrated into the partnership and federal exchanges. The result is a great deal of signal noise and chaos around how regular consumers and families will understand their options to increase their access to health care. There are also conflicting viewpoints concerning the potential outcomes of insurance exchanges. Some argue that certain benefits of the exchange may become its Achilles' heel—open enrollment, individual choice, and risk adjusters may promote incentives for adverse selection. Premiums and corresponding risk adjustments of premiums are examples of selection devices that may be used to discourage enrollment of certain populations within an exchange [5]. As implementation of the insurance exchanges unfolds at the state and federal level, one must monitor the potential adverse effects.

Previous experience implementing insurance exchanges also demonstrates the need to update research hypotheses and evaluation techniques to reflect unanticipated outcomes. Massachusetts was one of the first to experiment with a robust health insurance exchange, the Commonwealth Connector. This channel enabled people to compare private health plans and provided a means for eligible individuals to enroll in its public health insurance plan, Commonwealth Care. A report from the McKinsey Global Institute in February 2011 strongly suggested that the expansion of public health insurance and the development of a health insurance exchange for the individual market would eventually "crowd-out" employer-provided health insurance among working age adults [6, 7]. These concerns proved unwarranted as Massachusetts saw an increase in both the number of employer-sponsored health plans and the percentage of working age adults being covered by them [8].

The ACA further mandates that all qualified health plans, Medicaid non-managed benchmark or benchmark-equivalent plans, and plans offered in the state exchanges offer a minimum level of coverage, defined as the essential health benefits. Current law identifies 10 broad categories of mandated coverage and states that the scope of the benefits offered must equal those offered under a typical employer plan. The proposed rule goes further to outline four options that can be used as a state-specific benchmark plan. If one of the 10 benefit categories is not included in the benchmark plan, supplemental coverage must be offered [9].

Defining the essential health benefits has proven to be a socially charged endeavor. Patient and consumer advocates believe that this minimum benefit standard fulfills a promise of guaranteed health security to all Americans. And while many of these new protections receive widespread support, they will also be expensive. Thus, it is this conflict between comprehensiveness and affordability that throws into question the final framework of the essential health benefits. In an effort to mitigate the potential controversy, the Institute of Medicine Committee recommended that the Department of Health and Human Services (HHS) create a formalized board that uses evidence-based cost estimates to update the essential health benefits package [10]. Additional uncertainty stems from the guidelines released in November 2012, which grant states new authority in developing their own essential health benefits [11]. The essential health benefits may not have the far-reaching breadth originally envisioned as states use this power to dilute certain provisions [12]. As one example, states are only required to offer coverage for the *number* of drugs per category found in the state's benchmark plan. Consumers had hoped for a national definition of the essential health benefits and worry that benchmark plans may be adjusted to minimize coverage options.

The Basic Health Plan as an Access Point

The ACA also contains a significant provision that allows states to create a more affordable alternative to the health insurance exchanges, the Basic Health Plan. The ACA allows states to contract with a managed care plan to offer insurance coverage that includes the state's minimum essential health benefits. The Basic Health Plan would target those individuals and families with incomes between 133 and 200 % FPL or incomes just above Medicaid levels. In addition, legal immigrants within the 5-year waiting period would be eligible to apply for coverage through a Basic Health Plan.

The Basic Health Plan offers a cost-effective option for reducing the number of lower-income uninsured people, thus likely to be a financially and politically savvy option for states to consider. As a federally financed endeavor, states would receive 95 % of the federal money that would have otherwise been spent on premium tax credits and cost-sharing subsidies offered in the exchanges. The Urban Institute projects that states could recoup $1,000 per enrollee, savings that would then be reinvested in the Basic Health Plan in the form of increased provider rates or higher subsidies [13]. It also hopes to promote continuity of care and capture those beneficiaries who migrate back and forth between Medicaid and the health insurance exchanges. For consumers, the Basic Health Plan promises lower premiums and copayments than those sold on the exchanges [14, 15].

Despite the aforementioned advantages of the Basic Health Plan, states must assess how it will impact the viability of the exchanges. Roughly one-third of those eligible to access insurance through the exchanges, or 7.5 million individuals, would have income levels below 200 % FPL [13]. Smaller risk pools and greater administrative costs per beneficiary may challenge the self-sustaining aspect of insurance exchanges. And despite intentions to increase access to low-income individuals, capacity issues for Medicaid health plans and low provider reimbursement may translate into narrow provider networks for those insured by the Basic Health Plans [13, 15].

Political uncertainty has added further ambiguity as to whether states will adopt a Basic Health Plan. The Department of Health and Human Services has not released any significant guidelines that clarify federal funding or administrative costs. State decisions may be dependent on whether or not they pursue the Medicaid expansion. In some cases, federal matching rates may prove to be higher with the Basic Health Plan than with the Medicaid expansion. Conversely, implementing the Basic Health Plan may further fragment the already piecemeal healthcare system.

Bending the Cost Curve Through Innovations in Payment

Successfully implementing new payment models that incentivize coordination across the continuum, that have an increased focus on quality outcomes, and that encourage efficiency is critical to the success of healthcare reform. New models appropriately allow providers, payers, and patients to share in the savings and productivity gains that result from improved health and efficient resource utilization. The ACA espoused several new payment and delivery models, most notably bundled payments and accountable care organizations (ACOs). The Congressional Budget Office estimates that ACOs could accrue $4.9 billion in Medicare savings over 10 years while bundled payments for hospital and post-acute care could save Medicare closer to $19 billion in that same time. In total, payment and delivery systems that aim at improving the quality of care, appropriating services, and decreasing waste could save $418 billion in 10 years [16, 17].

Episode-based care, or bundled payments, is a reimbursement strategy that aggregates multiple fee-for-service payments into a single value. Providers are then reimbursed a flat fee for a clinically defined treatment or condition. Bundled payments reduce system waste by eliminating overutilization and duplication of services while also including bonuses for providers who reach performance and quality benchmarks. Medicare launched its first bundled payment demonstration in 2009 with the Acute Care Episode (ACE) Demonstration for Orthopedic and Cardiovascular Surgery. Prospective bundled payments were used to reimburse the participating organizations for selected orthopedic Medicare Severity Diagnosis-Related Groups (MS-DRGs) and/or cardiac MS-DRGs. Providers and hospitals participated in the gain-sharing program and there was an additional, atypical provision that allowed a percentage of the savings to be mailed directly to the beneficiary 90 days after discharge [18].

Early success from the Hillcrest Medical Center, one of the first to participate in the ACE demonstration, highlights the potential utility of episode-based care in payment reform. However, Medicare beneficiaries worried that they were being shortchanged on care as they received checks as part of the shared savings. The ACE demonstration shows how a reform that sounds wonderful in intention and design—and whose high-quality medical and financial results showed great promise—may have a different outcome in implementation and execution.

Although a single demonstration project does not form a basis for generalizing across the whole Medicare system, it does impart important lessons learned and instruct the implementation of future pilot programs. One such lesson was the importance of public education. Patients do not typically realize the extent to which change is necessary to align payments with high value care. Many assume that the financial incentives for physicians and other providers are already set up for proper care. If beneficiaries perceive, rightly or wrongly, that their doctors are withholding care, it will reverberate loudly throughout the system. Public education is therefore essential to implementing any health reform, specifically, that higher cost does not equate with better quality. Many experts are now exploring how physicians can better communicate with patients about right care and better care rather than more care. A number of experts have weighed in on this topic, including the Medicare Payment Advisory Commission, Center for American Progress, Brookings Institution, Catalyst for Payment Reform, and the Society for General Internal Medicine. Shared insight on this topic will be particularly relevant as Medicare launches its Bundled Payments for Care Improvement.

Accountable care organizations (ACO) have also been lauded as a means to improve health outcomes and the quality of care while slowing the growth of overall costs. Accountable care organizations bring together coordinated networks of providers with a shared responsibility to provide high value care to the patients. If an ACO can achieve quality targets while slowing the spending growth, it will share in the savings. The ACA calls for the development of several Medicare ACO pilot programs. As of July 2010, there are 256 organizations participating in the Medicare Shared Savings Program, Pioneer Program, or Physician Group Practice Transition Demonstration and over four million Medicare beneficiaries benefiting from the coordinated care of ACOs.

The Physician Group Practice Demonstration was the first Medicare initiative that offered incentives for physicians to collaborate on healthcare delivery and improve quality and cost efficiency. Early results from the PGP Demonstration illustrate the potential for both savings and quality improvements. Overall annual savings from the 10 participating physician groups was $114 per Medicare beneficiary and $532 per dual eligible. In addition, participants reported reductions in 30-day readmission rates and surgical readmission rates for dual eligibles [19].

The ACA established a pediatric ACO demonstration project. With deficiencies in pediatric care just as widespread as in adult care, the ACO concept is highly relevant [20]. Not only are children's health care costs among the most rapidly rising component of healthcare services, but current payment models do not reward efforts that improve child health outcomes [21]. Despite the success of the ACO model and its applicability to pediatric care, the specified starting time for the pediatric demonstration project has passed without any guidance from HHS. The lag in developing pediatric ACOs highlights the difficulty in implementing one pilot program across patient populations. The ACA must develop a process for using what is learned from one demonstration to inform the development of said program with different patient populations.

The Independent Payment Advisory Board (IPAB) is one opportunity to help transition successful pilot programs into broader policy. In an effort to reduce cost growth and improve the quality of care, the 15-member IPAB was commissioned to provide annual recommendations on changes in Medicare payment in years that Medicare spending was projected to exceed specified targets. These recommendations would become law if Congress did not propose an alternative proposal, thereby mitigating the influence of politics and creating a mechanism to move toward payment reform without congressional action. The IPAB also was tasked with submitting reports on general healthcare costs, quality, and access and recommending nonbinding strategies to slow the growth in private healthcare expenditures [22, 23]. The Center for Medicare and Medicaid Services (CMS) Office of the Actuary estimated that the IPAB could reduce Medicare costs by $24 billion in 10 years [24]. However, Republicans are steadfast in their opposition to the IPAB. Despite appropriating $15 million for the IPAB in 2012, little else has been achieved to advance implementation of the board.

Payment reforms aimed at benefit design, most notably value-based insurance design (VBID), have similarly experienced delayed implementation. Copayments and deductibles hold patients accountable for their healthcare decisions and help address the problem of overconsumption. Conversely, cost sharing can dissuade the use of preventive services that may have prevented the onset of disease. The VBID approach makes cost sharing a function of the clinical value of different services [25, 26]. A pilot program by Pitney Bowes in 2001 reduced copayments for drugs in a specified therapeutic class. While the lower levels of consumer cost sharing may have cost money at the start, Pitney Bowes was able to recoup those costs and generate additional savings through improvements in health. One year after implementation, Pitney Bowes reported $1 million in savings and significantly reduced emergency department utilization [25, 26]. The Medicare Payment Advisory Commission (MEDPAC) and HHS recognize VBID as an important strategy to promote high value care and the ACA has included specific legislation that encourages utilization of VBID [27].

Ultimately, the complexity of implementing some of these innovative payment reforms, cost containment measures, etc., will be dependent upon the other aspects of the ACA—access, quality, etc.

Improving Quality

The third core principle concerns the quality of care in our country—we know from McGlynn and colleagues that our care is appropriate or of good quality only about half of the time [28]. As a result, there is a great deal of waste and inappropriate care that only compounds the issues related to access and cost. Quality reporting initiatives are predominant in the ACA and they work to encourage transparency and promote better quality within the healthcare delivery system.

Medicare adopted a rather robust system of quality reporting for physicians, hospitals, and health plans. The Physician Quality Reporting System was first established in 2006 and uses financial incentives to encourage healthcare providers to report on the quality of care given to Medicare beneficiaries [29]. Originally a voluntary program, the ACA requires physician participation beginning in 2015. Medicare's Hospital Value-Based Purchasing Program will soon extend to outpatient surgery centers as CMS looks to implement a pay-for-reporting program in ambulatory settings in 2014. Health plans must also demonstrate how they utilize benefit design, value-based payment models, and other market-based incentives to encourage high-quality health care. More specifically, the CMS Innovation Center is bringing a new level of transparency to healthcare quality and performance measures with the Medicare Advantage STARS program. Those Medicare Advantage plans that receive scores of three stars or better, based on survey and administrative data, will receive bonus payments from Medicare [30].

The progress that has been made in Medicare until now has been overshadowed by the significant lag in applying a federal structure for quality measures to Medicaid. The variation in states' Medicaid programs and quality reporting initiatives makes application of a national Medicaid quality reporting program difficult. The target audience for each state plan has a unique set of needs that necessitates the use of different benefit designs or reimbursement features. State oversight, governance entities, employers, and providers add additional layers of complexity and variability [30]. As such, developing a federal structure for quality measures has proven more difficult than originally anticipated.

In an effort to create more commonality across states and programs, the ACA calls for the development of the Medicaid Adult Quality Measures Program. An initial set of healthcare quality measures for Medicaid-eligible adults was released by HHS in January of 2012. Efforts are also being made in the realm of pediatric care. The Department of Health and Human Services released a report in 2012 that showcases the progress made in systematically measuring and reporting on the quality of care children receive in Medicaid/CHIP [31]. CMS has made significant progress toward developing the Federal-State Data Systems for Quality Reporting, a model that will improve the quality of reporting by different states. A balance must be struck that supports uniform standards to foster benchmarking capabilities while also recognizing the diversity seen within the quality reporting realm. Developing the means to test and evaluate reporting measures on a regular basis will facilitate the creation and evolution of a dynamic federal reporting system.

Conclusion

Expanding access to health care while also reforming the payment and delivery system by linking provider reimbursements to quality metrics and total cost reductions are hallmarks of this new era of health reform. While the November 2012 election has secured the future of the ACA, have we achieved the aforementioned aims? Access to coverage for some of the most vulnerable populations is still in question as Republicans look to target certain provisions. In other cases, cost concerns have severely minimized coverage or benefit options. Moreover, real-world application of the law is subject to the dynamic and variable nature of the healthcare system. Past demonstration projects must be used to inform the necessary follow-legislation to assure that the original objective is achieved. The ACA can only be deemed a success when in 5, 10 years we've delivered on the promise of Medicare's triple aim of improving the experience of care, improving the health of populations, and reducing per capita costs of health care.

References

1. Jennings CC. Implementation and the legacy of health care reform. N Engl J Med. 2010;362(15):351.
2. Holahan J, Buettgens M, Carroll C, Dorn S. The cost and coverage implications of the ACA medicaid expansion: national and state-by-state analysis. The Urban Institute; November 2012. Available from: http://www.kff.org/medicaid/upload/8384.pdf
3. Estimates for the Insurance Coverage Provisions of the Affordable Care Act Updated for the Recent Supreme Court Decision. Congressional Budget Office; July 2012. Available from: http://cbo.gov/sites/default/files/cbofiles/attachments/43472-07-24-2012-CoverageEstimates.pdf
4. Summary: five basic facts on immigrants and their health care. Kaiser Family Foundation; March 2008. Available from: http://www.kff.org/medicaid/upload/7761.pdf
5. McGuire TG, Sinaiko AD. Regulating a health insurance exchange: implications for individuals with mental illness. Psychiatr Serv. 2010;61(11):1074–80.
6. Singhal S, Stueland J, Ungerman D. How US health care reform will affect employee benefits. *McKinsey Quarterly*; June 2011.
7. Employer survey on US health care reform: details regarding the survey methodology. McKinsey; 20 June 2011. Available from: http://www.mckinsey.com/features/us_employer_healthcare_survey
8. Long SK, Stockley K. Massachusetts health reform: employer coverage from employees' perspective. Health Aff. 2009;28(6):1079–87.
9. Essential Health Benefits Bulletin. Center for Consumer Information and Insurance Oversight; 16 December 2011. Available from: http://cciio.cms.gov/resources/files/Files2/12162011/essential_health_benefits_bulletin.pdf
10. Iglehart JK. Defining essential health benefits—the view from the IOM Committee. N Engl J Med. 2011;365(16):1461–3.
11. Obama administration moves forward to implement health care law, ban discrimination against people with pre-existing conditions. *News Release*. Department of Health and Human Services; 20 November 2012. Available from: http://www.hhs.gov/news/press/2012pres/11/20121120a.html
12. Levey NN. Passing the buck—or empowering states? who will define essential health benefits? Health Aff. 2012;31(4):663–6.
13. Dorn S. The basic health program option under federal health reform: issues for consumers and states. The Urban Institute; March 2011. Available from: http://www.urbaninstitute.org/UploadedPDF/412322-Basic-Health-Program-Option.pdf
14. Cassidy A. Basic Health Program. Health Policy Brief. Health Aff. 15 November 2012. Available from: http://www.healthaffairs.org/healthpolicybriefs/brief.php?brief_id=80

15. Bachrach D, Dutton M, Tolbert J, Harris J. The role of the basic health program in the coverage continuum: opportunities, risks and considerations. Kaiser Family Foundation and Manatt, Phelps, and Phillips, LLP; March 2012. Available from: http://www.kff.org/healthreform/upload/8283.pdf

16. Estimate of direct spending and revenue effects for the amendment in the nature of a substitute released on March 18, 2010. Congressional Budget Office; 18 March 2010. Available from: http://www.cbo.gov/publication/21351

17. Affordable care act update: implementing medicare cost savings. CMS Office of the Actuary. 2010. Available from: http://www.cms.gov/apps/docs/aca-update-implementing-medicare-costs-savings.pdf

18. Medicare acute care episode demonstration for orthopedic and cardiovascular surgery. Centers for Medicare and Medicaid Services. Available from: http://www.cms.gov/Medicare/DemonstrationProjects/DemoProjectsEvalRpts/downloads/ACE_web_page.pdf

19. Colla CH, et al. Spending differences associated with the Medicare Physician Group Practice Demonstration. J Am Med Assoc. 2012;308(10):1015–23.

20. Mangione-Smith T, et al. The quality of ambulatory care delivered to children in the United States. N Engl J Med. 2007;357:1515–23.

21. Children's health care spending report: 2007–2010. Health Care Cost Institute; July 2012. Available from: http://www.healthcostinstitute.org/files/HCCI_CHCSR20072010.pdf

22. Guterman S, Davis K, Stremikis K, Drake H. Innovation in medicare and medicaid will be central to health reform's success. Health Aff. 2010;29(6):1188–93.

23. Jost TS. The independent payment advisory board. N Engl J Med. 2010;363:103–5.

24. Estimated Financial Effects of the 'Patient Protection and Affordable Care Act,' as Amended. Centers for Medicare and Medicaid Services. Office of the Actuary; April 2010. Available from: http://www.cms.gov/Research-Statistics-Data-and-Systems/Research/ActuarialStudies/downloads/PPACA_2010-04-22.pdf

25. Chernew ME, Rosen AB, Fendrick AM. Value based insurance design. Health Aff. 2007;26(2):195–203.

26. Choudhry NK, Rosenthal MB, Milstein A. Assessing the evidence for value-based insurance design. Health Aff. 2010;29(11):1988–94.

27. The University of Michigan Center for Value-Based Insurance Design. Available from: http://www.vbidcenter.org

28. McGlynn EA, Brook RH. Keeping quality on the policy agenda. Health Aff. 2001;20(3):82–90.

29. Centers for Medicare and Medicaid Services. Physician Quality Reporting System. Available from: http://www.cms.gov/Medicare/Quality-Initiatives-Patient-Assessment-Instruments/PQRS/index.html

30. Hoo E, Lansky D, Roski J, Simpson L. Health plan quality improvement strategy reporting under the affordable care act: implementation considerations. The Commonwealth Fund; April 2012

31. 2012 Annual report on the quality of care for children in medicaid and CHIP. Department of Health and Human Services; December 2012. Available from: http://www.medicaid.gov/Medicaid-CHIP-Program-Information/By-Topics/Quality-of-Care/Downloads/2012-Ann-Sec-Rept.pdf

Chapter 4
What We Got (and What Might Have Been): A Distinctly American Approach

Shawn Bishop

The Affordable Care Act (ACA) is two pieces of legislation passed by Congress and signed into law by President Barack Obama in March 2010.[1] The first piece is the Patient Protection and Affordable Care Act (PPACA or "p-pocka" in inside-the-Beltway speak), to give the ACA its full and proper name. The second piece is the healthcare provisions of the Health Care and Education Reconciliation Act (HCERA), which amended certain elements of PPACA and works in conjunction with it.

Two bills to enact healthcare reform became necessary after Republicans in both the House and Senate opposed the Democrats' health reform efforts and candidate Scott Brown won the Massachusetts special election to fill the Senate seat vacated by the death of Democratic Senator Edward Kennedy. This special election occurred on January 19, 2010, in the middle of negotiations between House and Senate Democrats on a final version of the health reform law. The House had passed its initial version of health reform (the Affordable Health Care for America Act) on November 7, 2009, while the Senate had passed its initial version (the Patient Protection and Affordable Care Act) on December 24, 2009. Democrats in both the House and Senate were able to pass their initial versions of healthcare reform without support from Republican members as they held sufficient voting majorities in each chamber to do so. However, House and Senate Democrats still needed to negotiate differences between their respective health reform bills and then pass the negotiated version in each chamber in order to send a final version to the President.

Scott Brown's election ended the Democrats' 60-vote majority in the Senate, because as a Republican his vote would give Republicans the 40th vote they needed to use filibuster rules to block bills from proceeding to votes in the Senate. A filibuster is a historical method per Senate rules that allows 40 Senators to prevent final

---

[1] P.L. 111-48 and P.L. 111-52.

S. Bishop, M.P.P. (✉)
Marwood Group, Washington, DC, USA
e-mail: sbishop@marwoodgroup.com

H.P. Selker and J.S. Wasser (eds.), *The Affordable Care Act as a National Experiment:*   27
Health Policy Innovations and Lessons, DOI 10.1007/978-1-4614-8351-9_4,
© Springer Science+Business Media New York 2014

action (i.e., a floor vote) on a bill for any length of time without consequence.[2] Therefore, with 59 and not 60 votes, Senate Democrats no longer held a sufficient majority to avoid the use of filibuster on a final version of health reform that they would negotiate with the House. However, Senate rules also exempt one type of bill from the use of a filibuster: a budget reconciliation bill whose provisions only serve to decrease or increase the federal deficit. Such a bill must meet specific Senate criteria to be deemed a reconciliation bill. Once the criteria are met, a reconciliation bill can proceed to a Senate vote under regular order where a simple majority (i.e., 51 votes) can secure passage. Thus, Democrats in Congress had a way to pass a final healthcare reform bill that could avoid Senate filibuster if (1) the House passed the initial Senate version of health reform, PPACA, and (2) both chambers then passed their negotiated changes to PPACA in a stand-alone reconciliation bill. The Health Care and Education Reconciliation Act of 2010 contains the negotiated changes amending a handful of provisions in PPACA. Once both chambers of Congress passed PPACA and HCERA, they had created the final version of the health reform law that the President could sign.

The combination of PPACA and HCERA comprises 10 titles, approximately 456 provisions, and 907 pages of consolidated print. Figure 4.1 shows the number of provisions and consolidated pages in each of the 10 titles. Medicare and coverage expansion have the most provisions and the most pages.

With its hundreds of provisions, the ACA, as the combined bills have come to be known, does many things. Through titles I and II, it expands health insurance coverage to millions of Americans through a combination of public and private sources. It prohibits insurance practices that have kept consumers from obtaining or affording health insurance coverage in the private market. For example, it prohibits insurers from denying coverage for preexisting conditions, from charging women higher premiums than men, and from charging elderly consumers more than three times the premium they offer to younger consumers. It provides insurance subsidies for individuals with lower incomes and small employers with less than 50 workers. It creates insurance markets, or exchanges, in each state where individuals and small groups can compare health insurance plans with objective information and apply for federal subsidies in a one-stop shopping environment. It imposes penalties on individuals who have access to affordable health insurance coverage but do not carry it (i.e., the individual mandate) and on employers (with 50+ workers) who do not offer affordable health coverage (i.e., the employer penalty) to their employees.

Title III reduces the growth rate in Medicare payment rates for most services. It changes payment and care delivery in Medicare through new incentives and requirements for providers and physicians to deliver safer, more coordinated and efficient care to their patients. A large but lesser-known part of the ACA, Title VI, significantly expands authority to reduce fraud, waste and abuse in Medicare and Medicaid. Almost 200 of 900 pages in the bill are devoted to redressing fraud, waste and abuse alone.

---

[2] The Senate filibuster rules can be used to delay or indefinitely block a bill from ever moving to a floor vote. Once bills have proceeded to floor votes, the rules under both the House and Senate allow them to secure passage with a simple majority (i.e., 51 votes).

Vital Statistics of the Affordable Care Act (ACA)

➤ **ACA is a combination of two pieces of legislation**

   1) Patient Protection and Affordable Care Act (PPACA)

      • Passed by the Senate on December 2009 and passed by the House on March 2010

   2) Health Care and Education Reconciliation Act of 2010 (HCERA) which modified PPACA

      • Passed by the House on March 2010 and by the Senate on March 2010

➤ **Comprises 10 titles, 456 provisions, and 907 pages of text**

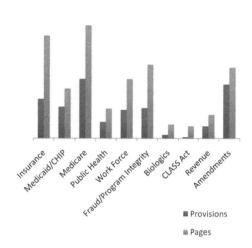

Fig. 4.1 The ACA is comprised of multiple legislation, titles, and provisions totaling 907 pages. (Source: based on analysis from the Marwood Group Advisory, LLC, 2012)

Title IV of ACA provides new authority and funds for public health programs. For example, it creates a $15 billion (since reduced by Congress by over $6 billion) "Prevention and Public Health Trust Fund" to help states and communities promote wellness and prevent disease, while Title V extends programs and funds for training of medical professionals, including physicians, nurses, and nurse practitioners. Title VII establishes authority for the approval of generic versions of biologic drugs, which use living organisms to treat diseases such as cancer. Title IX imposes new excise taxes on health-related manufacturers and health insurers and higher Medicare taxes on individuals with higher incomes to help pay for expanding coverage and public health activities. Other parts of ACA establish programs for new long-term care insurance options (Title VIII) and make amendments to other provisions of the bill (Title X). If we step away from the main titles and look for the major themes in the bill, we can see that healthcare delivery system reform comprises the bulk of the bill in terms of the number of pages and the number of provisions in it. Almost 70 % of both the number of pages and the number of provisions are devoted to the healthcare delivery system (Fig. 4.2). Sheer number of pages or provisions does not necessarily equate to public policy impact in any given piece of legislation. But in the ACA, it is a clear indication of an intentional effort by Congress to focus on reforming the delivery of care through provisions that establish new payment models for delivering care, new organizational models and tools for delivering care,

Delivery System Reform Provisions Comprise Bulk of ACA

➢ When grouped into thematic parts, provisions addressing
  delivery system reform comprise bulk of the health reform bill

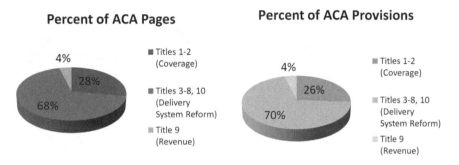

Fig. 4.2 The majority of pages and titles in the ACA deal with delivery system reform. (Source: based on analysis from the Marwood Group Advisory, LLC, 2012)

programs to train the healthcare workforce, new approaches to delivering preventive care for chronic disease, new research about what works in medicine, and other reforms. Many but not all of ACA's delivery system reforms are initiated through the Medicare and/or Medicaid programs. Nevertheless, Congress intended them to influence as appropriate the delivery of care in the health system writ large, i.e., for all patients including those covered by their employers in the private sector or other federal programs.

A focus on delivery system reform is not new in terms of federal legislation. Congress introduced the topic of paying Medicare providers for quality rather than volume in the Medicare Modernization Act of 2003 and the Deficit Reduction Act of 2005, for example. What is different about the ACA is the breadth and intensity with which it attempts to reform the delivery of care in the US that no recent efforts, legislative or otherwise, have done. Certainly the extension of medical coverage to the poor and elderly through Medicare and Medicaid in 1965 had and will continue to have enormous impact on the US health system. While the enabling legislation was historic in establishing a binding social commitment, its focus was providing coverage and payment under the delivery system that existed at the time, not in reforming the system of care.

Moreover, the ACA uses a distinct approach to delivery system reform. In what follows I highlight three features of the approach taken by ACA that, from my perspective as a former health committee staffer to Chairman Max Baucus of the Senate Finance Committee as the bill was being written, are remarkable compared to other federal health laws of modern times. The ACA has been controversial since its inception, and others who were close to its development will have their own views. But pro or con, many will agree that ACA's approach to delivery system reform has distinctive features.

So what is distinctive? First, the law takes the goals of improving quality and protecting patients as the rationale for delivery system reform, as suggested by the Institute of Medicine over 10 years ago in its watershed report, *Crossing the Quality Chasm*. Patient safety is a major theme and undercurrent throughout the entire bill. As the full name of the law—the Patient Protection and Affordable Care Act—suggests, it is the primary purpose. The ACA ramps up improvements in the safety of care for patients through payment-related incentives and new requirements for providers and physicians to initiate better modes and processes of care under the Medicare and Medicaid programs, which are large enough in terms of patients and healthcare spending to serve as levers that instigate change in the healthcare system as a whole. Key provisions in the bill, for example, reduce Medicare and Medicaid payment to hospitals if too many of their patients are readmitted within 30 days or acquire infections. For the first time in history, federal programs covering 80 million lives will financially reward hospitals that keep patients safer and penalize hospitals that do not. These provisions are intended to encourage hospitals to improve the way they deliver care to all patients and are already being adopted by payers in the private sector.

These reforms are just two of many examples of how the ACA seeks reform of the delivery system through improvements in care. The ACA also reduces Medicare payments to facilities (such as hospitals and post acute care providers) and private plans (i.e., Medicare Advantage plans). Those savings were included to reduce overpayments that the nonpartisan Medicare Payment Advisory Commission recommended to Congress. But Congress also for the first time links a portion of Medicare payments to hospitals and health plans practitioners to the quality of care they deliver. This link reflects Congress' view that while payment reductions on their own reduce program spending, they are rarely catalysts for needed improvements in the delivery of care. Many members of Congress would have liked to avoid blunt Medicare payment reductions in the ACA. Instead the bill would have paid for expanding health coverage solely by making large-scale improvements in the delivery of care. Unfortunately, the Congressional Budget Office (CBO), Congress' official scorekeeper of the budgetary effect of legislation, could not certify sufficient savings from care delivery changes alone to cover the costs of expanding coverage. One reason is CBO only scores effects of legislative proposals on federal spending. To the extent ACA improves care and lowers costs outside of federal health programs, those savings are not counted. Another reason is that even though Congress included numerous ideas that were believed or known at the time to improve safety and quality of care, CBO perceived some of those ideas to have cost neutral effects, i.e., no federal savings. Even though CBO did not score improving care with large savings, Congress persisted in making those changes its primary approach to delivery system reform in the ACA.

The ACA's insurance coverage expansion also protects patients because it will reduce dangerous gaps in care that individuals with no insurance coverage often face. Numerous studies have shown that having health insurance improves health outcomes, such as better life expectancy and fewer complications from chronic disease. Health insurance exchanges can be seen as another form of patient protection because they will facilitate comparisons of insurance benefits so patients can choose plans that fit their medical needs, provide ratings of the quality of care delivered by health insurance plans so consumers can choose ones that deliver better care, and transfer federal subsidies to health insurers so that gaps in coverage and care will be less common. According to CBO, about 25 million Americans will obtain coverage through exchanges by 2022. However, ACA's coverage expansion is not projected to produce full universal coverage, so there will still be risk for gaps in care for some Americans.

Second distinctive feature of ACA's delivery system reforms is that it begins to turn the US health system away from fee-for-service medicine. Reducing the amount of health care paid on a purely fee-for-service basis (by testing bundled payment models, for example) is not a new idea. Payers in the private sector have been putting in place or testing similar changes. But as a matter of principle, the ACA adds weight of Medicare spending to some initial steps toward turning the US health system away from paying on a fee-for-service basis.

Members of Congress had heard from health services and medical research communities that much of what is wrong with the US health care in terms of poor quality and high costs can be traced back to incentives in delivering care under fee-for-service arrangements. ACA establishes for the first time payment under Medicare and Medicaid for "accountable care organizations" composed of physicians and providers who choose to work together and use technology to deliver coordinated care to their patients. These organizations will be financially rewarded if they deliver high quality and lower cost care on a population basis, which provides incentives to deliver cost effective care and not just more care as under fee for service. ACA also creates pilots to pay hospitals under bundled rather than fee-for-service payments. And although many criticize the ACA for not doing more to reform or eliminate fee-for-service payments, the ACA provides new forces that can be built upon to help move the system in that direction.

Third distinctive aspect of the ACA is that it seeks to make delivery system reform self-sustaining. Congress added provisions to the bill, such as the Center for Medicare and Medicaid Innovation (CMMI), whose purpose is to test, evaluate, and then *apply* payment and care delivery changes that lower costs while maintaining or improving quality in these programs.

Members of Congress said they would like progress in healthcare delivery system reform not to be fully dependent on their being able to pass a bill. To date, no employer or health insurance plan in the US has had enough clout or resources to initiate systemic reform on its own. As a result, reform of the US health system has been stalled or conducted in a piecemeal fashion because it needed to be initiated through legislation from Congress. The need to extend statutory authority to apply reforms has put needed progress in healthcare delivery in a precarious spot.

Congress not only created the CMMI but also capitalized it with $10 billion every 10 years. That is, CMMI is authorized to invest $10 billion every 10 years in experiments in payment and care delivery as more is learned about the effects of ACA reforms and more is learned about new ideas that might work. Through CMMI, Medicare and Medicaid can provide an ongoing platform for innovation in healthcare delivery, with funding that automatically renews. CMMI will first test new ideas for payment and care delivery. If those ideas work, then the Secretary of Health and Human Services (HHS) has authority to apply them on a nation-wide basis in those programs without having to gain additional approval from Congress. That is a distinctive feature of the ACA.

The ACA also establishes the Patient-Centered Outcomes Research Institute (PCORI), whose purpose is to improve health and healthcare decision-making by patients and providers by comparing the clinical effectiveness of existing medical treatments. The ACA funds PCORI's research activities with $4 billion over 10 years. Unlike CMMI, PCORI will need to be reauthorized to continue beyond 2019. PCORI was not central to insurance market reform. But it reflects foresight on the part of Congress that if the US health system was going to trend away from fee-for-service toward accountable care, then more evidence on what works or does not work in health care would be needed. Finally, the ACA also requires for the first time the Secretary of HHS to establish national priorities for improving the safety and quality of care and to measure progress in the US health system toward them. Every year, HHS will issue a report that measures the quality of health care in the US and tracks progress toward the national goals. Setting goals and measuring progress will help inform providers, researchers and policymakers of new areas that may need attention. Even though the ACA is extensive and multifaceted in scope, there were items left out. Major pieces of legislation rarely include all provisions that were considered. Some are left behind because the policy is not fully mature; others are left behind because political consensus is lacking. One example is reform of cost sharing for Medicare beneficiaries. Cost sharing includes deductibles, copayments, coinsurance, and premiums to help cover the costs of Medicare coverage. Ways to change cost sharing had been proposed in the past, but the ideas were not fleshed out in time for consideration. In addition, higher cost sharing in the form of increased deductibles or copayments did not have enough political support at the time to be fully considered. Higher premiums to be deducted from beneficiaries' Social Security payments were too controversial to be included in the ACA. Given these limitations, the ACA focused on changes that lower Medicare spending by improving care and reducing overpayments to providers and health insurance plans. The bill made no changes to medicare cost sharing for medical services and no negative changes to benefits. In fact, the ACA added preventive benefits at $0 cost sharing and reduced cost sharing for prescription drug benefits under Medicare. But given the rate of growth in the number of Medicare beneficiaries and in total spending for the program in the coming decades, there will be a need to consider changes to cost sharing. The Medicare Payment Advisory Commission is working on principles and policy options for Congress to consider. It is very likely that Congress will have a discussion about Medicare cost sharing as it grapples with how to reduce the federal deficit.

   Another idea left on the table is value-based benefit design either in Medicare or the new health insurance exchanges. Value-based benefit design is related to cost sharing in that it attempts to set it in ways that encourage the choice of treatments, providers, and lifestyle behaviors that lead to appropriate and cost-effective care. It can take many forms, such as the development of tiered networks that would differentiate cost sharing based on the cost and quality performance of providers. For instance, patient cost sharing would be set lower for higher quality, lower cost providers and higher for lower quality, higher cost providers. Changes to the tax preference for health benefits also was a policy looked at by the Senate Finance Committee. Allowing employers to exclude healthcare benefits from taxable wages is a tax expenditure that amounts to over $200 billion in foregone revenue to the US Treasury each year. Making changes to this tax policy also proved too controversial at the time to be fully considered by Congress. However, like cost sharing for Medicare beneficiaries, the tax preference for employer-provided health benefits will likely be reconsidered in the context of serious deficit reduction talks that are expected to occur over the next several years.

   Those are examples of what did not make it into healthcare reform. But what might have been? What alternative to the ACA could have Congress passed? One answer is a bill to expand health coverage for kids only. The then-White House chief of staff Rahm Emanuel pressed Congress to move toward a kids-only package on the grounds that it would be less controversial and take less time to craft and pass. As a presidential candidate in 2008, then-Senator Obama had health insurance for all children as part of his campaign platform. But most Democrats in Congress were not convinced that young adults, working poor and their families with no health insurance from their employers, and near elderly who live without insurance coverage should be left behind if they were going to go through the effort to develop and negotiate a bill.

   A kids-only bill might have been easier to pass. It may have garnered a few Republican votes. But we would have had none or few of the delivery system reforms that will improve care for all patients in the US, no help addressing problems in fee-for-service payment, no self-sustaining provisions for delivery system reform, and no distinctive way of reforming the American healthcare system that future efforts can look upon.

References

1. Call to Action: Health Reform 2009. White Paper prepared by Senate Finance Committee Chairman Max Baucus, November 12, 2008.
2. Estimates for the Insurance Coverage Provisions of the Affordable Care Act Updated for the Recent Supreme Court Decision. Congressional Budget Office, July 2012.
3. Estimates of Federal Tax Expenditures for Fiscal Years 2011-2015. Joint Committee on Taxation, January 17, 2012.

4. Dorn S. Uninsured and Dying Because of It: Updating the Institute of Medicine Analysis on the Impact of Uninsurance on Mortality. The Urban Institute; 2008. Available from: http://www.urban.org/publications/411588.html
5. Avanian JZ, et al. Unmet health needs of uninsured adults in the United States. JAMA. 2000;284(16):2061–9.
6. Roundtable to Discuss Reforming American's Health Care Delivery System, United States Senate Committee on Finance, April 21, 2009. Available from: http://www.finance.senate.gov/hearing/?id=d85e499a-01ed-23b6-7c6e-a200e6bee498

Part II
Don't Get Mad, Get Data: Conducting the Experiment

Chapter 5
Commentary on Part II: Conducting the Experiment

Brian Rosman

As the hoary, misquoted aphorism from PoliSci 101 goes, states are "laboratories of democracy."

The sentiment is correct, but the actual phrase comes from a 1932 dissenting opinion by Supreme Court Justice Louis Brandeis. Oklahoma required ice distributors to get a license from the state. The Court majority overturned the law, ruling that there was nothing distinct about ice distribution that allowed a state to limit competition. Brandeis disagreed and, with the background of a severe national economic depression, argued that this economic regulation should be permitted: It is one of the happy incidents of the federal system that a single courageous state may, if its citizens choose, serve as a laboratory and try novel social and economic experiments without risk to the rest of the country.

For many decades, the Commonwealth of Massachusetts has been a laboratory for social and economic experiments in health care. Since the 1980s, the state has tried a dramatic health policy endeavor once a decade. Each of these experiments influenced national policy.

In 1988, under Governor Michael Dukakis, it enacted far-reaching legislation establishing universal health coverage. The centerpiece of that law was the policy of "pay or play," requiring most employers to either "play," provide health coverage to their workers and families, or "pay," pay an assessment to the state equal roughly to the cost of providing family coverage, which in turn would be used to provide subsidized insurance.

While the pay or play provisions of the law were never implemented, and ultimately repealed in 1996, the Dukakis law included a number of other policy experiments that influenced national policy, including expanded coverage for children, subsidized coverage for people with disabilities who are working, and funding health coverage for people receiving unemployment benefits. Another provision

B. Rosman, JD. (✉)
Health Care For All, Boston, MA, USA
e-mail: rosman@hcfama.org

H.P. Selker and J.S. Wasser (eds.), *The Affordable Care Act as a National Experiment:* *Health Policy Innovations and Lessons*, DOI 10.1007/978-1-4614-8351-9_5,
© Springer Science+Business Media New York 2014

required all college students to have health insurance, the first instance of a state individual mandate. All of these provisions remain in Massachusetts state law today.

Then, in 1996, the state overhauled its Medicaid program. The program was renamed "MassHealth," with greatly expanded eligibility, a simplified application process, and most members enrolled in managed care systems. The expansion was facilitated by a generous deal worked out with the federal government, using the Medicaid waiver process to allow Massachusetts to claim additional federal funds. Section 1115 of federal Medicaid law, inspired by the spirit of the Brandeis dictum, allows state "Research and Demonstration Projects" that test new ways of providing health coverage to low-income people.

Using the Section 1115 process, the Clinton administration allowed Massachusetts to claim federal Medicaid funds for expanded coverage and support for safety-net hospitals that went beyond traditional Medicaid limits. This waiver was renewed several times. But as budgets grew tight and the George W. Bush administration looked critically at the waiver coming up for renewal in 2005, Massachusetts was facing a crossroads, and Governor Romney had to act.

Many factors converged to lead to the passage of the 2006 reform law, known in the state as "Chapter 58," as it was the 58th law enacted that year. (Note that while the law is now popularly known nationally as "Romneycare," no one called it "Romneycare" until there was an "Obamacare.") Among the key forces leading to the law were:

- First, the number of uninsured in Massachusetts had been growing since the 2001 recession. While the 1996 Medicaid expansion was successful in driving down the number of uninsured (from around 680,000 to 365,000), by 2004 the number of uninsured people had grown to about 460,000 people.
- Second, with the growth of the uninsured came increased demands on the state's Uncompensated Care Pool, a hospital reimbursement program funded by hospitals, insurers, and the state. The program was designed to require minimal state funding, around $30 million. But growing numbers of uninsured patients showing up at hospitals led to increased state funding, reaching $206 million in 2006. Another $56 million in costs was unfunded in 2006 and thus absorbed by hospitals.
- Third, the Blue Cross and Blue Shield of Massachusetts Foundation had begun a major research project, called the Road Map to Coverage. The project looked at coverage expansion options and provided cost estimates of various reform plans.
- Fourth, a broad coalition of healthcare groups, organized by advocacy nonprofit Health Care For All, formed to push for coverage expansions. The coalition, known as ACT! (Affordable Care Today), included the state's hospital association, medical society, community health centers, and numerous influential civic and religious groups. A subset of ACT! gathered some 140,000 signatures to place a reform plan on the ballot, with the intent to force legislative action. The ballot measure was pulled once Chapter 58 was enacted.
- Fifth, the federal government had signaled that it was no longer willing to renew the MassHealth waiver without changes. By 2006, the waiver was providing the state with over $350 million in federal funds for the state's safety-net hospitals.

- Sixth, Governor Mitt Romney was interested in finding a market-oriented approach to covering the uninsured. His staff had consulted with the Heritage Foundation, a conservative Washington think-tank. They had advised him on a number of ideas that had also informed the early-90s Senate Republican alternative to the Clinton plan, centered around an individual mandate, a structured market for coverage, and sliding-scale subsidies for private insurance.

These concerns coalesced in the legislative process that led to enactment of Chapter 58 with virtually unanimous majorities in both the House and Senate. Governor Romney signed the law, with Senator Edward Kennedy looking over his shoulder, in the historic Faneuil Hall, with Romney campaign TV crews capturing the whole thing for anticipated use in Romney for President TV ads.

The elements of the law included further expansion of MassHealth (Medicaid), mainly for children; sliding-scale insurance subsidies for low- and moderate-income adults (Commonwealth Care); a reformed individual health insurance market, with an exchange, called the Health Connector, to make it easy to compare and purchase plans; and requirements on employers to offer and individuals to obtain coverage, if it's affordable.

As implementation began in fall 2006, nobody knew precisely how the experiment would turn out. The state relied on a sophisticated econometric simulation model, prepared by Massachusetts Institute of Technology economist Jonathan Gruber, to forecast impacts on premiums, employer reactions, and coverage expansions. Gruber was also named to the Health Connector board, where he could play a further role in monitoring implementation. But the model was only as good as its input data and assumptions, both of which were not assured.

Six years later, Massachusetts' former Secretary of Health and Human Services, Dr. JudyAnn Bigby, presented the results of the Massachusetts experiment. In her chapter, Dr. Bigby explains the key policy initiatives contained in Chapter 58 and reports on the results. The health reform law expanded coverage substantially, encouraged more employers to offer coverage, lowered premiums for individuals, was affordable to the state, and improved the overall health of the population.

In her chapter, Dr. Bigby presents a blizzard of statistical data showing the impact of the Massachusetts law. Population coverage increased by 439,000. The uninsurance rate decreases by 1.9 %. Over 100,000 more children are covered. Minority adults with a usual source care increase from 84 % to 91 %.

But statistics only tell part of the story. At Health Care For All, we connect these statistics to the thousands of real people whose lives have been improved because of health reform legislation. For some, their lives have literally been saved because of the availability of affordable health coverage. Through our toll-free helpline, we hear every day from Massachusetts residents. Several case studies are offered as examples (names have been changed):

1. Ana and Ben never thought about the value of health insurance. When health reform was passed and they learned that every resident of Massachusetts needed to have health insurance, they signed up for MassHealth and Commonwealth Care. Right after enrolling, Ana became pregnant with their first child. Their

baby, Matthew, appeared at first to be a health child. But, after regular checkups, the doctors diagnosed the baby with a very rare cancer. The doctors found tumors in his brain and lips as well as an enlarged liver, three times larger than in an average baby. Ana and Ben were devastated. Ana and Ben thought their little son's life would probably end.

Right away Matthew started chemotherapy and intense cancer treatment. For four months they were living at the hospital every day. Matthew surprised everyone who thought that he wouldn't make it, even some of his physicians. Now he is two years old and his parents say that he really enjoys life. They say that playing with his friends and eating ice cream are his favorite things in life.

2. Janet enrolled in Commonwealth Care about two years ago. She was completely caught by surprise when her eyes felt watery, with a feeling like there was sand in them. It continued to worsen, and she started to see spots, have extreme irritation, swelling, sensitivity to light, and pain. All of these symptoms occurred over three days.

Because of her coverage, as soon as she felt ill, she immediately went to the doctor. The initial diagnosis was a virus, but the medicine did not work. A more complete eye examination diagnosed her eye problem as uveitis, a rare inflammation in the middle layer of the eye. She soon had the proper medicine needed to treat the disease. Janet says that she is just so grateful about all the professional care she had because uveitis can lead to permanent blindness.

She wrote, "I'm just so lucky to be a Massachusetts resident. I just can't imagine what I would do if I had to pay out of pocket for my doctor's visits and medicine. I think that we only realize the value when something bad really happens to us. Health is just so fragile. Anything can happen anytime and we definitely need to be prepared to take care of ourselves."

3. Thomas realized the importance of having access to health insurance after he suffered two strokes in the same year. He says that he never liked going to the doctor, and in his mind he would never need to see one. But when the stroke hit, Thomas was brought to an emergency room by one of his teenage daughters. At the time he worried that it would cost him so much that probably he might never be able to afford to pay for all the medical expenses.

That's when Thomas learned about the health coverage offered by the state to low-income uninsured people. Soon after, Thomas was notified about his Commonwealth Care eligibility and could continue his treatment to prevent any kind of serious stroke from happening again. Since then he has been taking medicine. Thomas said having been so close to death, he now knows that having the access to affordable health insurance is something vital for every human being. Here is what he had to say:

> I almost thought I would die, or maybe have my life completely changed having to live like a vegetable. I still can see the looks in my daughters' faces when they saw me at the hospital. We all thought that I wouldn't be able to make it. But thank God, MassHealth helped me in all the best way to make it possible for me to be treated by great professionals at a wonderful institution.

4. Amanda contacted Health Care For All when she found out that she was unexpectedly pregnant. She was uninsured and had no idea how she would afford prenatal treatment, as well as the delivery costs. She was notified about her eligibility for Healthy Start, which is a MassHealth program that covers every eligible pregnant woman. Her Healthy Start coverage made it possible for Amanda to get all of the necessary prenatal treatments, and her son, Eric, was born healthy.

But two months later and after several exams, Amanda learned that she had a brain tumor. Fortunately, Amanda learned about her health condition just in time for treatment. She says she is so lucky to be a Massachusetts resident and to have the chance to get the best care she could ever have covered by an affordable healthcare coverage plan.

The success of Massachusetts' reform, in both the statistical and human dimensions, demonstrated the importance of the Affordable Care Act (ACA or, of course, "Obamacare"). The Obama administration and congressional bill writers looked to the experience of Massachusetts in formulating policy. Economist Jonathan Gruber and other Massachusetts policy gurus shuttled back and forth from Boston to Washington, explaining the unfolding impact of the Massachusetts reforms to federal policymakers.

As explained in the chapter by Bruce Landon of Harvard Medical School and Stuart Altman of Brandeis University, the ACA is built on the same policy foundations as the Massachusetts reform, but with differing details:

1. An expansion of Medicaid eligibility to low-income people
2. Sliding-scale tax credits to reduce the cost of private insurance
3. Exchanges in every state to facilitate the purchase of coverage by allowing comparison of plans that meet minimum standards
4. Insurance reforms, by ending preexisting-conditions exclusions and other practices that shut people out of coverage
5. An individual mandate, requiring everyone to purchase coverage if it's affordable
6. An employer responsibility provision, requiring large employers to offer coverage to their workers

Landon and Altman are optimistic about the ACA, in large part due to the success of Massachusetts reform. They conclude that "While there is much that is unknown about the impact of the ACA, lessons from Massachusetts and other experiments in payment and delivery reform suggest that most Americans stand to benefit from its passage."

With the new decade of the 2010s, Massachusetts was again due for another far-reaching healthcare experiment. In summer 2012, the legislature enacted a far-reaching bill (known as Chapter 224) aimed at controlling cost growth. The law's major planks include increasing care coordination, using payment incentives to promote health and efficient care, and investing in public health prevention programs. The law also includes transparency provisions, malpractice reforms, expanded primary care, and many other features. Altman and Landon also discuss this reform, which takes some of the suggestions, demonstrations, and pilot projects in the ACA and expands them to statewide mandates.

While Massachusetts gets lots of attention, other major statewide health policy experiments are occurring. The most dramatic is unfolding in Vermont, where the building blocks are being put in place for moving to a government-funded, single payer, universal coverage health system in 2017. In 2011, the legislature voted to begin a planning process to bring all health care under the state's umbrella. The law also included a charge to regulate the health delivery system to promote health and reduce costs. The most difficult decisions, on how to finance the plan, were delayed until after the reelection of the supportive Governor, Peter Shumlin. Governor Shumlin was handily reelected in 2012 on a platform of support for the single-payer plan, and now the process is moving forward.

Leading the work is Anya Rader Wallack, chair of the Green Mountain Care Board which oversees the reform project. In her chapter, Rader Wallack details how data is driving Vermont's reforms, and how that data can inform federal policy as well.

As the Massachusetts policies mature in the next few years, the Vermont experience may provide new inspiration for those following in Brandeis' footsteps, seeking "novel social and economic experiments" at both the state and federal level.

Chapter 6
The Affordable Care Act as an Experiment: Data We Have, Expect to Have, and Should Have, from a Vermont Pilot Study

Anya Rader Wallack

The federalist governmental structure of the United States gives the 50 states a huge role in implementing many national policies. Nowhere is this more the case than in health care. For example, although the federal government administers Medicare with one set of rules for the whole country, the 50 states each separately administer Medicaid with their own rules as long as they meet certain federal criteria. This has been so since the inception of the two programs in 1965. The Affordable Care Act (ACA) likewise has blanket nationwide provisions while also giving each state responsibility, if it so chooses, for implementing key aspects of the law. For example, states may establish and operate their own health insurance exchanges under the ACA, or they may default to a federal option. Even if states choose not to operate health insurance exchanges, the ACA enables states to do lots of other things in terms of healthcare innovation and creates new relationships between the federal government and state governments around issues, such as insurance reform, where they previously haven't had much of an interface.

With regard to insurance reform, the ACA sets a nationwide standard for carriers who until now have been almost entirely regulated at the state level. It also institutes new regulations for the small-group and non-group insurance markets that some but not all states established beginning in the 1990s. The ACA has thus created a new floor for insurance coverage that extends across all states. This remains true despite the Supreme Court's overturning of the ACA's attempt to expand Medicaid, a ruling triggered by a suit filed against this provision of the law by 26 state attorneys general.

By the middle of 2012 a dozen states had passed legislation to operate their own insurance exchanges under the ACA. It remained to be seen how many other states might join them in doing so.

A.R. Wallack, Ph.D. (✉)
Green Mountain Care Board, Montpelier, VT, USA
e-mail: anya@arrowheadha.com

H.P. Selker and J.S. Wasser (eds.), *The Affordable Care Act as a National Experiment:*
Health Policy Innovations and Lessons, DOI 10.1007/978-1-4614-8351-9_6,
© Springer Science+Business Media New York 2014

Thus, if we look at the Affordable Care Act as an experiment, we've got a lot of variation across states and therefore, as with many other federal policies that allow for variation across states, not a particularly well-controlled experiment. I think nonetheless there are things that we can do to compile the data we will need at both the state and federal level to understand the before and after of the ACA and the continuing impact of its policies and to generalize about groups of states, individual states, and the United States in general.

In terms of the variation across states, there are a couple of areas that are particularly important. One is that the states have many different starting points. States like Massachusetts and Vermont, for example, have long had many of the insurance reforms called for in the ACA. Massachusetts, which passed a near-universal health insurance coverage law in 2006, instituted a number of important reforms beginning in the mid-1980s. Likewise Vermont, where I serve as chair of the Green Mountain Care Board, which the Vermont legislature established in 2011 to oversee health reform in the state, passed community rating and guaranteed issue for the small-group market in 1991 and followed that with community rating and guaranteed issue for the non-group market in 1993. Guaranteed issue means that insurance carriers cannot deny coverage to potential customers based on their risk profile—their age, gender, health status, occupation, or other factors that might affect their healthcare costs. Community rating means that health insurers are limited by law in the extent to which they can charge higher rates (premiums) for people who, for example, are predicted to use more health care based on their age, gender, health status, or occupation.

Our early implementation of guaranteed issue and community rating has had an impact on how many carriers we have in our market, the kind of carriers, and their rate differentials. Currently, in Vermont, we have three carriers doing business in the commercial market. Only two of those offer coverage on the small-group and non-group markets.

This creates a very different environment than in states such as Mississippi, Texas, or Utah. These and in fact, most other states have not experienced, or faced the prospect of, such measures in their insurance markets prior to the ACA.

States are also in very different places in terms of coverage and coverage policy. The extent to which their populations are covered by employer-provided insurance varies tremendously from state to state. The states in the Northeast tend to have a lot of employer coverage, and this coverage tends to be fairly generous compared to the national average.

The extent to which states have used Medicaid as a platform to maximize coverage also varies a great deal. States like Massachusetts and Vermont have used Medicaid creatively to cover as much of their populations as possible. That's not true across the country for a variety of policy, financial, and political reasons.

Last but not least, states are also in very different places in terms of healthcare data availability and their ability to use that data to maximize outcomes under the ACA. We can begin to get a sense of that by considering the overarching goals of the ACA:

- Consumer protection
- Coverage expansion

- Expanded preventive and primary care
- Reduced disparities
- Increased provider efficiency and quality
- Reduced cost growth

If we think about the evaluations that might be desirable relative to these goals, various experimental designs could apply. But any experimental designs we can envision would require large amounts of data—big data, in the jargon of our day.

The ACA created some new data sources at the federal level to track these kinds of things. This is particularly so in terms of the interface between the states and the federal government on insurance regulation. We've seen some of this play out already in terms of the medical loss ratio requirements at the federal level, with the feds now having data that says what's happening at the state level with carriers in terms of their loss ratios and rate increases. In addition, states will continue to report to the federal government on Medicaid programs the same way they have in the past.

But in large part, states seeking to maximize outcomes under the ACA will rely on data sources that predate the law's drafting and enactment in 2009–2010. The best data that are being brought to bear in terms of measuring the ACA are in states that were pursuing a health reform agenda before the law came to be. These states—not only Massachusetts and Vermont, but Minnesota and other states—had already beefed up their data efforts to provide more regular data feeds, better data collection capacity, and to some extent better analytic capacity in order to track their own progress irrespective of the ACA.

There will be new data reporting around the state-operated health insurance exchanges. Some of that is still to be defined, and I think to a great extent, states will be left to decide what kind of data collection, analysis, and reporting they want to do for their own purposes. There is not a strong federal framework here.

Some states are collaborating on these issues through the State Health Access Data Assistance Center (SHADAC), a program of the Robert Wood Johnson Foundation and a part of the Health Policy and Management Division of the University of Minnesota School of Public Health. SHADAC works to develop cross-state approaches to health data collection and analysis, and it is developing a common framework for evaluation of implementation of the ACA. But again, there aren't strong requirements for this at the federal level.

The data the federal government will likely find most useful to evaluate progress against the ACA's goals include:

- National and state surveys of changes in the numbers of people insured, uninsured, and underinsured after implementation of the law
- Healthcare Effectiveness Data and Information Set (HEDIS) findings by state and state/federal surveys on preventive and primary care
- Expenditure and cost driver trends
- Workforce coverage
- Population group disparities
- Provider quality and efficiency

There are some things that will happen at the federal level around provider quality and efficiency as a result of the payment reform experimentation and new policy implementation that the ACA includes. There are national surveys to track the uninsured and to some extent the underinsured, and there are state surveys to complement the federal ones. But the important point here is once again that there is as yet no strong national framework in place to collect, analyze, and disseminate the relevant data.

This means we're going to continue to see a lot of state variation. Some states will have very good reporting about what's going on and a very good sense of what the impact of the ACA is, and I believe that Vermont is an example of where that might happen.

Vermont is aggressively implementing the ACA. We see the ACA as a way of advancing a lot of policy goals that we have at the state level. We actually see the ACA as a platform for going beyond what it establishes and requires.

There are a couple of things that we see as particularly advantageous to us in the ACA. One of them, of course, is money. The ACA brings money to Vermont in the form of federal tax credits for people who will get coverage through the exchange and receive a tax credit to lower the cost of their health insurance. It also brings money to Vermont to rebuild infrastructure in our Medicaid eligibility system and in the health information technology systems that are critical to any kind of broad-based simplification of health insurance.

Vermont Governor Peter Shumlin has an agenda of moving towards single payer health insurance coverage in the state, and we are using the Affordable Care Act as part of our effort to achieve that goal. We want to cover the entire Vermont population through a very simplified uniform system. We passed a bill in 2011 to create our own health insurance exchange, as provided for in the ACA, and we're using ACA money to build it.

To date we are the only state in the nation to require that the small-group and non-group markets purchase insurance through a state exchange, and this will start in 2014. From then on there will be no outside of the exchange purchases for those markets. Folks will purchase through the exchange, and it will be to the greatest extent possible a seamless system for people who are purchasing private insurance with no subsidy, people who are purchasing private insurance with a new tax credit, and people who are on public programs.

We're really trying to marry together the public and private, and as part of that scheme we are also the only state in the country to put the exchange in our Medicaid agency. In some states, that would be a strange idea. But in Vermont the distinction between public and private sometimes becomes less meaningful.

We also plan to apply for a federal waiver under the ACA so that we can decouple the insurance financing coverage from employment. But we can't receive that waiver until 2017 at the earliest under current federal law. In the meantime we'll be setting up an exchange and operating under the same rules that all other states are operating under.

The 2011 bill establishing these policies and actions also set up the Green Mountain Care Board, which I mentioned at the beginning of the chapter. The

Green Mountain Care Board's purview is concerned with improving the quality of individual care and population health, constraining the rate of growth in state healthcare costs, and reforming payment systems in ways consistent with those objectives.

In those senses the Green Mountain Care Board reflects at the state level the goals of the ACA at the national level. However, to say that does not quite capture the scope and aims of the board. In the Green Mountain Care Board the state of Vermont has created a statutory authority that really goes beyond the ACA in terms of both its regulatory role and the extent to which we are pursuing payment reform across all payers, public and private.[1]

My colleagues and I on the board have very broad authority we can implement, including oversight of health insurer rates and hospital budgets. Soon we will have purview over hospital capital expenditures. We intend to do a lot of evaluation of our efforts at the state level, and a lot of that will be very consistent with the kinds of things that the federal government would want to measure.

If Vermont is an example of a state that loves the ACA, then New Hampshire offers a really nice contrast that is literally right next door (Figs. 6.1 and 6.2). The two states have a lot in common. We're both into maple trees and maple syrup. We've both got covered bridges, although theirs are bigger. In terms of how they look on the map, I always say New Hampshire's upside down, and in New Hampshire they probably say Vermont's upside down. We are very similar states in terms of the nature of our populations, their lack of diversity, the percentage of rural versus urban residents.

At the same time we are very different states politically. Right now in New Hampshire, it's almost illegal to talk about the ACA. They are not trying to implement the act, and they will be relying on a federal fall back rather than a state health insurance exchange. As a result, even though there is some really good data in New Hampshire around health care and they've done a lot of the same kind of work that we've done in Vermont to build up their health-related datasets, I expect New Hampshire will not soon make an active effort to use its data to evaluate things related to the ACA.[2]

To step back from a New England close-up and consider the national scene, there are as I said earlier a dozen or so states that have pursued exchanges and a whole lot of states that were not yet doing anything as of mid-2012. After the November 2012 elections, some of the latter states began to show more interest in implementing health exchanges and other parts of the ACA. With the end of the election cycle, officeholders in and from these states would likely want to pursue a share of the very large amount of federal dollars that the ACA has put on the table, and this is continuing to evolve (Fig. 6.3).

---

[1] In this regard I might note that by some third-party measures, Vermont has the best health care in the country (see Fig. 6.7). This is not necessarily an unalloyed good. It can encourage complacency and prevent us from setting the bar as high as we can and should.

[2] In fairness to my neighbor state, I should note that it also occupies a high ranking in third-party assessments of health-care quality (see Fig. 6.7).

Vermont loves the ACA!

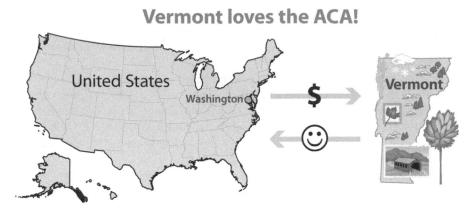

Fig. 6.1 Vermont loves the ACA!

New Hampshire? Not so much!

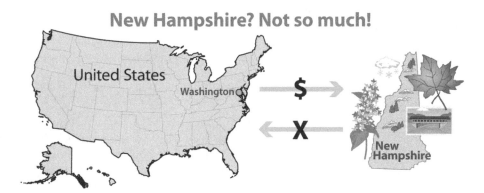

Fig. 6.2 New Hampshire? Not so much

If we want to get details of state-to-state variations across the country, we run into some serious challenges. For example, the Commonwealth Fund has tracked the variation in the uninsured rate across states, and there are a number of data sources that can be used for measuring who's insured and who's uninsured (Figs. 6.4 and 6.5).

The first main challenge in using these data is that they tend to be old. If you want to know what happened last year in terms of coverage in your state, seldom are the data up to date enough to help you with that. As we in Vermont much more aggressively pursue policies that are related to the ACA, the timeliness of our data is a real challenge. Knowing what happened two years ago or three years ago isn't good enough for assessing the impact of legislative and policy changes.

Another challenge for small states like Vermont or Rhode Island is that in national surveys the sample size at the state level is so small that it's either

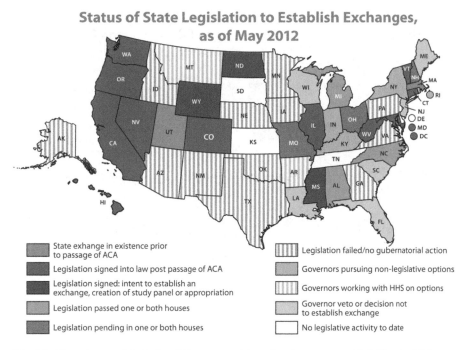

Fig. 6.3 There is a great deal of variation across states when it comes to establishing health insurance exchanges (Source: National Conference of State Legislatures, Federal Health Reform: State Legislative Tracking Database. Available from: http://www.ncsl.org/default.aspx?Tabid=22122; Politico.com; Commonwealth Fund analysis)

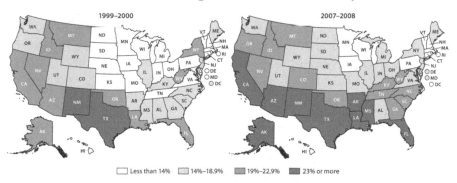

Fig. 6.4 Since 1999, there has been a substantial increase in the number of insured adults (Source: Commonwealth Fund State Scorecard on Health System Performance, 2009)

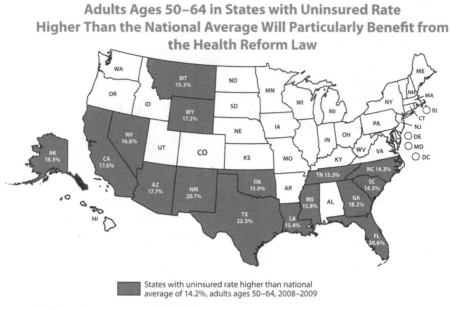

Fig. 6.5 Certain states, particularly in the south, have the highest number of uninsured adults and will therefore benefit most from ACA expanded coverage (Source: Analysis of the March 2009 and 2010 current population survey by N. Tilipman and B. Sampat of Columbia University for The Commonwealth Fund)

meaningless or so volatile from year to year that it's very hard to track anything. So even if you can get it on a more up-to-date basis, you can't trust the data until you have multiple years accumulated and you're looking at larger trends instead of narrow year-to-year trends.

Vermont is striving to secure more detail, and there are similar efforts in some other states. We use data from a variety of sources, including a state level household telephone survey that we have done in the past on either an annual or every other year basis. Then we supplement from other data that we get through our regulatory processes either from insurance carriers or other sources that we use to build an annual Vermont healthcare expenditure analysis.

We look at the full array of coverage within our state, and this ends up being a much better source of information for a small state like Vermont. You can't look at something like the Bureau of Labor Statistics' and Census Bureau's joint Current Population Survey (CPS) and understand with this granularity what's going on in Vermont. But when we try to get below this level, which shows that there's 250,000 people in Vermont who are covered through insured products, we don't always have the kind of information that we'd like to have about who's insured, what kind of groups they're in, how their rates vary, and how their products vary. So we're doing a lot of work in Vermont to understand more about what happens within each of these slices.

2009 State Scorecard Summary of Health System Performance

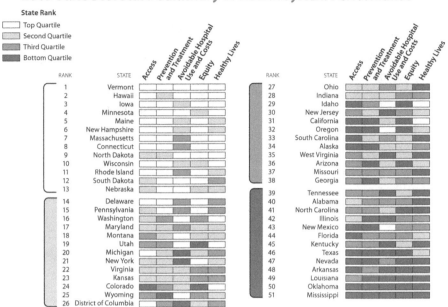

Fig. 6.6 2009 state scorecard summary of health system performance (Source: Commonwealth Fund State Scorecard on Health System Performance, 2009)

Going back to the overarching goals of the ACA, there are sources for varied types of data that can inform our evaluation of progress towards those goals. The Commonwealth Fund has again probably done the best job of summarizing data across states on some of these other dimensions that have not been measured particularly well on a state-by-state basis in the past (Fig. 6.6).

The Commonwealth Fund data provide state-by-state insight into access to care, prevention, and treatment; avoidable hospital use and costs; healthcare equity and disparity for vulnerable population groups; and healthy lives in general. The data are of high quality, but for a small state you'll often see small numbers that reflect a small sample size and that are somewhat out of date.

Data from 2009 might not sound that old. But in the case of a state like Vermont, where we're trying to look at things like avoidable hospital use and prevention in the context of our payment and delivery system reform initiatives and fine-tune those initiatives as we go, these data are too limited and too old. They don't provide the recent and current detail that we need to make reasonable policy decisions. We have to collect better data ourselves with our providers, and we are spending a lot of effort in Vermont right now figuring out what kind of data collection we're going to do and how we are going to evaluate our success.

That will never roll up to this kind of national dataset that allows for state-to-state comparison. On the other hand, the kind of work that SHADAC does where they bring together some of the states that have been most active on these fronts may allow for that kind of comparison over time.

The problem is that it is very expensive to conduct a statewide survey, and it is disproportionately expensive for a small state like Vermont to contact enough of its population to obtain adequate data. Of course, to do a national survey that had a big enough sample for Vermont would be very expensive, too. One way or another, somebody's got to pay to call enough Vermonters. A model for us here is another of our neighbor states in New England, Massachusetts, which has been a real leader in state-based data collection.

What we are trying to do in Vermont is follow federal definitions, particularly around the quality stuff and efficiency, so that we're not driving people crazy and we're allowing for benchmarking against other states and against national or regional norms. Our data collection priorities are:

- Surveys of Vermonters for time-relevant, robust-sample data on:

  - Coverage
  - Access to care
  - Patient experience and similar consumer-based measures

- Accurate, updated reporting from healthcare providers on:

  - Expenditure trends
  - Provider quality and efficiency
  - Expansion and meaningful use of health information technology
  - Provider supply
  - All-payer claims data

The last item, an all-payer claims dataset, is really critical to our efforts and to the efforts of at least 10 other states. All-payer claims datasets are state-mandated datasets to which insurance carriers must submit claims data. In the Vermont case, we require that all carriers submit claims data to state government, which is housed in a data warehouse and made available for research purposes. These datasets are in various stages of development in other states.

Vermont's all-payer claims dataset has been in place for five years. Up until this year, however, it was comprised of private insurance claims. We've just integrated Medicaid into that dataset, and we're in the process of integrating Medicare. It has required an immense amount of work to get data use agreements for everybody in place and to work through the complexities of combining private and public payer data. Other states, such as Minnesota, have been working through the same issues. Unfortunately, I think every state doing this has had to go through a tough development and learning process. But the good news is that a dozen or so states are developing really good claims data that we will be able to benchmark and compare across state lines. We still have a ton of work to do to share our experiences across states about how to analyze claims data, how to mush together Medicare, Medicaid, and commercial payers, and so on and so forth. But it's an exciting prospect that I believe will come to fruition over the next few years.

Healthcare researchers and other stakeholders can accelerate progress towards this goal by continually asking states like Vermont and Massachusetts, "When can we get the data, when can we get the data?" In the absence of researchers pressuring us to make those data available, we will take our time, because there are lots of other things to do, and release of the data requires review processes that are complicated. But I think we're going to end up getting some of the best analysis out of these datasets when researchers can take them and do analyses that we might never think of doing, or might simply be unable to do, at the state level.

What could the federal government do to help this along for the benefit of the country as a whole in implementing the ACA and achieving its goals, as well as for the benefit of individual states like Vermont that want to maximize the impact of the ACA within their borders and even go further? The answer in a nutshell is that we need standard measures across all states, and that is where the federal government must take the lead.

It's kind of scary when states start inventing measures all on their own. We do it for the best of reasons, but it really leaves us in a vacuum. You can sink a whole lot of resources into measurements that give you no basis for analyzing the comparative effectiveness of what you are doing in relation to what other states are doing against which you have no comparisons. So standard measures at the federal level are important.

The federal government could also give the states a big helping hand by moving closer to real-time release of Medicare data and easing restrictions on the states' use of the data. It's really hard to get Medicare data on a timely basis, and then it's four times harder to secure permission to do anything with that data.

One of the key things the states in the all-payer dataset group want to do with Medicare data is benchmarking. The federal government should not only allow this; it should encourage, facilitate, fund, and even require benchmarking across states with Medicare, Medicaid, and other healthcare data.

The states don't have the capacity or authority to do this on their own. Look again at the variations in coverage in the Commonwealth Fund's state-by-state healthcare scorecard (Fig. 6.6). What's behind those variations? How much are they the result of underlying factors for which we're not adjusting? If we in Vermont want to compare ourselves to other states that have very different politics and very different demographics, how do we do that?

The likelihood that any state, little or big, can accomplish that out on its own is slim. The federal government and the states will have to work together to achieve the clarity of data we all need to make the ACA as an experiment a successful one for the respective states and the nation as a whole.

The process is already well under way, albeit moving at different speeds in different states. As that process gathers momentum, we can imagine an array of perhaps a dozen data points, all central to the goals of the ACA, which we can track across the entire country, providing timely, accurate, well-adjusted state-by-state data that would allow everyone to know how they were doing (Fig. 6.7).

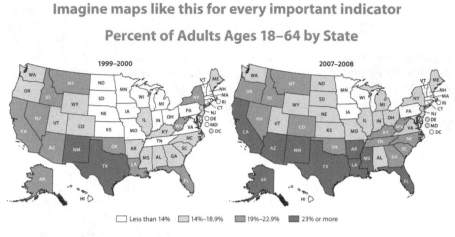

Fig. 6.7 We need to adequately measure important health indicators across the country (Source: Commonwealth Fund State Scorecard on Health System Performance, 2009)

For the moment, maps like this for every important indicator are a dream. But in the not too distant future, they can become a reality that will make an essential contribution to better healthcare in America and in each of the 50 states.

Chapter 7
The Center for Medicare and Medicaid Innovation: Its Purpose, Processes, and Desired Outcomes

Harry P. Selker

No other part of the Affordable Care Act (ACA) was more explicitly intended to serve as an experimental platform for the improvement of healthcare delivery than the Center for Medicare and Medicaid Services Center for Medicare and Medicaid Innovation, known as CMMI or the CMS Innovation Center. It was given an appropriation of $10 billion for use between fiscal years 2011 and 2019. According to the ACA statute, "The purpose of the Innovation Center is to test innovative payment and service delivery models to reduce program expenditures under the applicable titles [Medicare, Medicaid, and the Children's Health Insurance Program (CHIP)] while preserving or enhancing the quality of care furnished to individuals under such titles. In selecting such models, the Secretary [of Health and Human Services] shall give preference to models that also improve the coordination, quality, and efficiency of health care services furnished to applicable individuals..."

The idea behind the CMS Innovation Center is that, having had for many years a healthcare payment system that rewards greater volume rather than greater quality and greater efficiency, we now need to discover payment mechanisms that can improve quality and reduce costs.

The fundamental approach at the CMS Innovation Center, whether paying for primary care, hospital care, health systems care delivery, or state care, is to create a business context for innovation and to reward better quality and more efficiency. This context is intended to lead to a national healthcare system that improves the health of patients and reduces total costs.

A novel and very important feature related to the CMS Innovation Center is that if it conducts a test that demonstrates a new payment approach and reduces cost

H.P. Selker, MD, MSPH (✉)
Tufts Clinical and Translational Science Institute, Tufts University, Boston, MA, USA

Institute for Clinical Research and Health Policy Studies, Tufts Medical Center,
Boston, MA, USA
e-mail: hselker@tuftsmedicalcenter.org

H.P. Selker and J.S. Wasser (eds.), *The Affordable Care Act as a National Experiment:*
Health Policy Innovations and Lessons, DOI 10.1007/978-1-4614-8351-9_7,
© Springer Science+Business Media New York 2014

while maintaining or improving quality, it does not have to go through the usual Federal law-making process. Once the results are certified by actuaries, the evaluation can be brought to the Secretary of Health and Human Services who can make that payment approach national policy immediately. This is truly a unique opportunity to test and rapidly scale to a national implementation new payment approaches with the goal of improving quality and reducing costs.

Since the CMS Innovation Center began its work in 2011, it has been able to mount a wide array of programs in the field in several key categories. One is coordinated care, and that includes Pioneer and Advance Payment accountable care organizations (ACOs) and primary care initiatives. Another category pertains to "right care" during episodes in the hospital or transitioning out of the hospital. Another area relates to improving innovation infrastructure. A major focus is on the patients known as "dual eligibles," those eligible for both Medicare and Medicaid. This includes an interest in preventive care that is expected to increase substantially over time.

All projects in these areas are subject to rapid cycle evaluation and research, with findings disseminated by the CMS Innovation Center Learning and Diffusion team. The intent is not to do a test on only one type of provider or in only one type of setting. Rather, the goal is to hit the whole spectrum and to create incentives that have the potential to realign the way care is being delivered at all sites along the continuum of care. This could start in a very small practice site funded through an Innovation Award and then move to specific hospitals, then to larger groups of primary care doctors, then to health systems in ACOs, to "Pioneer ACOs," or to entire states for some of the CMS Innovation Center's dually eligible activities.

The Pioneer ACO model is one of the central initiatives in the category of Coordinated Care. The goal is to test the transition from a shared savings payment model to population-based payment. This was designed for healthcare organizations and providers that are already experienced in coordinating care. These are leaders in the field that are focused on improving the health and experience of care for individuals, improving population health, and reducing the rate of growth in healthcare spending.

CMS is publicly reporting performance data from 32 Pioneer ACOs, which can be found on the CMS website. For all of the models, CMS is providing participants with regular data feeds as well as performance feedback reports, on at least a quarterly basis. These data, in most cases, include not only the performance of the providers within the model but also performance on key healthcare quality metrics of competing providers outside the model. This will give participating providers a better sense of their performance against themselves historically and against others in the marketplace.

The Advance Payment model is based on the same approach, but in areas, such as rural USA, where having the needed initial capital is a barrier to starting an ACO. The goal in this case is to provide seed resources, in the form of advance payments, to enable more healthcare providers to start ACOs. The participating ACOs may receive upfront fixed payments, upfront payments based on the number of Medicare patients served, or monthly payments based on the number of Medicare patients.

The Comprehensive Primary Care Initiative is an experiment in seven healthcare markets, some statewide and some more localized: Arkansas, Colorado, New Jersey, the Capital District-Hudson Valley Region of New York, the Cincinnati-Dayton region of Ohio and Kentucky, the Greater Tulsa Region of Oklahoma, and Oregon. The goal of this program is to test a multi-payer initiative that fosters collaboration between public and private healthcare payers to strengthen primary care. It requires investment across multiple payers, because for a primary care doctor getting sums of money from Medicare but taking care of patients who are insured by a whole host of other different insurers, it is very difficult to allocate the funds to transform the practice to deliver the kind of services that ultimately a transformed primary care practice should deliver. That could involve, for example, hiring a nurse practitioner or investing in better health information technology.

Medicare's initial payments to healthcare providers in this program are approximately $20 per beneficiary per month. To incent lower costs, the program calls for shared savings for primary care doctors who deliver high quality care for lower cost. Where financial savings can be demonstrated by actuarial evaluation, CMS will share those savings with the primary care doctors while lowering the payments per beneficiary per month. Data are flowing to and from the seven test markets, each of which has approximately 75 practices and anywhere from three to 10 payers, including Medicare and private insurance plans.

A similar program that started even before the ACA, which was the impetus for the Comprehensive Primary Care Initiative, is the Multi-Payer Advanced Primary Care Practice (MAPCP) demonstration, although the specifics of the funds being provided are a little different. It is state-based rather than market-based, taking place in eight states: Maine, Vermont, Rhode Island, New York, Pennsylvania, North Carolina, Michigan, and Minnesota. As with the Comprehensive Primary Care Initiative, the idea is that providing upfront payment to primary care doctors will enable them to make the right kind of investments to transform their practices to deliver high quality care at lower cost.

The CMS Innovation Center is making a similar investment in Federally Qualified Health Centers (FQHCs). The impetus is to help FQHCs achieve a National Committee for Quality Assurance (NCQA) level three rating. The program follows essentially the same process as in the Comprehensive Primary Care initiative and MAPCP demonstration. Five hundred federally qualified health centers have been selected to participate, and the first performance year started November 1, 2011.

Under the Right Care initiatives, CMS Innovation Center is doing many things focused on acute care episodes. Partnership for Patients is a $1 billion investment with very ambitious goals to reduce preventable hospital-acquired conditions by 40 % over three years and reduce 30-day readmissions by 20 %—and thus save $35 billion—over the same period. In the first year after this was announced, nearly 4,000 hospitals signed the pledge; over three-quarters of the hospitals in the US are participating.

There are two major parts to this program. One devotes $500 million to improving patient safety. The safety part is testing intensive programs to provide training, support, and technical assistance to hospitals in making care safer. The CMS

Innovation Center has established and implemented a system to track and monitor hospital progress towards obtaining quality improvement goals, including engaging patients and families.

The Partnership for Patients ultimately aims to develop a learning network encompassing all of the participating hospitals. The CMS Innovation Center is aggressively trying to identify evidence from specific sites where there are hospitals that are doing well, where they are somehow able to improve quality and reduce costs. The Innovation Center is trying to identify the key features about these hospitals, and why they are successful, and then share the lessons across all the other hospitals.

The goal is to be able to harvest and spread the most effective strategies that are being used as quickly as possible. The intent is to disseminate the best evidence as part of creating a rapidly evolving environment in which there is mutual learning and continuous improvement.

The other half of the $1 billion Partnership for Patients is the Community-based Care Transitions Program. This also is a $500 million investment to reduce 30-day hospital readmissions, but this money is being made available to community-based organizations that handle patients' care after they leave the hospital. This could be in a post-acute care setting; it could be under the care of their primary care doctor. The goal is to reduce readmissions for high-risk beneficiaries and to document measurable savings to the Medicare program.

The central program that was recently announced is the implementation of bundled payments to promote care improvement. In the 1980s, CMS created diagnosis-related groups (DRGs) to bundle the payments of the hospital portion of inpatient hospitalization. Although not without shortcomings, most observers agree that it has been an effective mechanism to reduce the growth of costs of hospital care.

At that time, the physician portion was not bundled, and there remain many opportunities for physicians to try to maximize billing for the professional portion of hospital care. Similarly, in post-acute care settings, there are incentives aligned with billing as much as possible. Thus, the idea is to create a bundled payment for multiple services that a patient receives during a given episode of care. The Innovation Center is testing bundled payments for the services a patient receives during an acute care hospital stay alone, the acute stay and related post-acute care, or during post-acute care alone and will assess prospective as well as reconciled payment approaches.

In addition, the Innovation Center is investing in infrastructure to support more innovation. The Health Care Innovation Awards were announced in June 2012, with a total commitment of over $900 million, with individual awards ranging from $1 million to $30 million. The intent is to support a broad range of innovative service delivery and payment models to improve quality and reduce costs. This includes infusing capital into valuable ideas that are hard to get up and running. Evidence of how this has captured the attention of the healthcare community and systems is that CMS received close to 8,000 letters of intent to apply and close to 3,000 applications. Suggesting the potential for transformation, the Innovation Center found that these applications, almost without exception, included groups working with their direct competitors, often archrivals in their marketplace. Yet in these applications they were thinking about how they can share data and collaborate to improve care and reduce costs for the patients whom they serve.

This is seen by CMS as potentially one of the most useful aspects of the Innovation Awards. It appears that many projects that did not get funded by CMS are still moving ahead because these participants are talking to each other and recognizing the potential benefits to them of breaking down barriers in order to collaborate to improve quality and reduce costs.

In the Innovation Advisors Program, the Innovation Center is training individuals, many of them physicians, but also many pharmacists and other healthcare workers, to build continuous quality improvement programs in their respective institutions and organizations. Those who take part in the program get opportunities to deepen their skill sets in healthcare economics and finance, population health, systems analysis, operations research, and quality improvement.

The Innovation Center is devoting a great deal of effort to promoting more integrated care for dual eligibles, patients who receive both Medicare- and Medicaid-funded care, which generally previously has not been integrated. The idea is to understand how to integrate these sources of funding in order to have a cohesive approach for best managing these very vulnerable and very high-cost beneficiaries.

By mid-2012 15 states—California, Colorado, Connecticut, Massachusetts, Michigan, Minnesota, New York, North Carolina, Oklahoma, Oregon, South Carolina, Tennessee, Vermont, Washington, and Wisconsin—had received CMS contracts for demonstration models of integrated care for dual eligible individuals. Many of these models will be statewide, although some will not. Most will include capitated payment with the state, CMS, and a health plan entering into three-way contracts. Others will use a managed fee-for-service model, with the state and CMS entering into an agreement whereby the state can benefit from savings resulting from integrated care. The goal will be to bring these sources of support together to provide a coordinated way of managing the health of these very sick and vulnerable patients.

In the area of prevention, the Million Hearts Campaign aims to prevent a million heart attacks. It's focusing on diet and exercise, use of aspirin, blood pressure control, cholesterol management, and prevention of tobacco use.

A critical piece in the CMS Innovation Center is the Rapid Cycle Evaluation Group. Its job is not to sit on the sidelines and wait until the end of a demonstration to determine if an initiative did or did not work. Rather, its job is, on a very regular basis, to get data to participating healthcare providers to tell them how they are doing and how their competitors are doing, to create an environment where they can learn and improve. It is understood that there will be no turnkey solutions in any of these programs. Every one of these is going to require learning and evolution, and it is the central mission of the CMS Innovation Center to be part of that.

The Innovation Center understands that speed is crucial, but that it also cannot sacrifice rigor. It is understood that a lot of taxpayer dollars are at stake, and so investments must be made very wisely. There are many challenges in this, especially given the large number of programs that are going on simultaneously, but the

Center is using the most advanced epidemiologic methods and is building very sophisticated approaches in order to determine whether or not these programs are saving money while being quality neutral or better. Then the CMS Learning and Diffusion team helps share what was learned with providers in the field.

The ultimate goal is the development of a learning collaborative that brings together healthcare providers and payers in the interest of the nation's health and well being. Already in its early work, there is consensus that the CMS Innovation Center is making very significant progress to achieving that goal.

Chapter 8
The Dream of a National Health Information Technology Infrastructure

Craig Brammer

The ACA offers new, unprecedented opportunities to rethink the way health care is organized, delivered, and paid for. New payment models provided for within the Act, for example, are already helping to shift reimbursement approaches from fee for service, which incentivizes higher volume and intensity of care, to those that reward value.

Approaches such as accountable care organizations (ACOs), bundled payments, and medical homes seek to control the cost of health care by incentivizing more coordinated, efficient care that maintains patient health and avoids unnecessary expenditures.

However, modernizing the health sector requires the deployment of a more advanced information technology infrastructure. While other sectors of the economy have leveraged technology to drive dramatic improvements in productivity and consumer value for many years, health care has historically been slow to the party. Until recently, for example, most physicians relied on handwritten notes stored in file folders to maintain their patient records.

Importantly, the ACA was preceded by the Health Information Technology for Economic and Clinical Health or HITECH act. Designed to stimulate the adoption of health information technology (IT), HITECH included significant incentives for eligible hospitals and providers, along with a variety of programs to advance the field.

The activities of the Office of the National Coordinator for Health Information Technology (ONC), which was established within the US Department of Health and Human Services in 2004, ultimately seek to support the three-part aim of better health care, better health, and lower per capita costs. The ONC precedes the ACA, but the office and the legislation are natural partners with the same goals.

C. Brammer (✉)
HealthBridge, Cincinnati, OH, USA
e-mail: cbrammer@healthbridge.org

H.P. Selker and J.S. Wasser (eds.), *The Affordable Care Act as a National Experiment:* *Health Policy Innovations and Lessons*, DOI 10.1007/978-1-4614-8351-9_8,
© Springer Science+Business Media New York 2014

It's the belief of ONC and the Centers for Medicare and Medicaid Services (CMS) that echnology (and HITECH) forms the foundation for the new payment and delivery models we need to achieve the three-part aim, and the ACA has many provisions that express the same belief.

So what are the why, what, and how of HITECH? This Act helps to offset the cost of adoption of electronic health records. It enables providers to securely and efficiently exchange patient health information to ensure that providers have the right information at the right time to offer their patients the right care. It gives consumers tools to access their health information so that they can better manage their own health. And it's foundational to building a truly twenty-first century healthcare system where we pay for the right care, not just more care.

The basic building block for all of this is the concept of "Meaningful Use" of health information technology. As the ONC defines it, Meaningful Use is using certified electronic health record (EHR) technology to:

- Improve quality, safety, and efficiency and reduce health disparities
- Engage patients and family
- Improve care coordination and population and public health
- Maintain privacy and security of patient health information

Meaningful Use is driving the IT industry in ways that haven't happened before. And it is simultaneously incenting providers to adopt systems that will help achieve the triple-aim goals.

To increase Meaningful Use, the ONC is promoting standards and interoperability. It's stimulating innovation. And, in partnership with CMS, it's helping providers adopt electronic health records. It really is a national conversation that includes leading IT experts, but also clinicians from across the country in both rural and urban settings.

Stage 1 of Meaningful Use was about utilizing technology to gather information and jumpstarting the transition from paper to digits. Stage 2 is focused on care coordination, information exchange and operability, and patient access to data.

Ultimately stage 3 will bring health IT together with the concept of accountable care and models for improving care coordination. The point of all this is not the technology but, using technology to gather information, improve access to information for both providers and patients, and fundamentally transform care for the better.

The promise of electronic health records has been around for quite some time. But there has been a market failure that precluded the rapid adoption of electronic health records where the benefits of technology accrue to patients and those who pay for care but not always to those hospitals and physician practices who were expected to purchase the technology.

In the past few years, the adoption of electronic health records has been speeding up, thanks in large part to pilot projects and programs funded by CMS and ONC.

The momentum is definitely accelerating. The ONC goal for calendar 2012 was to have 100,000 eligible providers engaged in Meaningful Use of health IT. In June 2012 the number passed 110,000. Likewise when the ONC was started 2004, fewer than 1 % of physicians were e-prescribing. In 2012 over 70 % of physicians were e-prescribing. And most of that growth has occurred since 2008.

HITECH included funding for the ONC's Beacon Community Program. This "innovation fund" has become one of the country's most important means for testing health IT initiatives and determining which ones should be scaled up across the country. The program represents about $260 million, and the 17 Beacon Communities, each of which is receiving $12 million to $16 million over three years, represent regions across the country that had previously made significant progress in the adoption of health IT.

The Beacon Community Program goals include building and strengthening a health information technology infrastructure; improving health outcomes, care quality, and cost efficiencies; and spearheading innovations to achieve better health and health care. These Beacon Communities are microcosms of the rest of America, and, as such, the lessons that are learned from them will play a key role in healthcare transformation.

They range from Maine to Hawaii and from healthcare markets dominated by big, integrated providers like Intermountain Health Care in Utah, the Mayo Clinic in the upper Midwest, and Geisinger in central Pennsylvania to disaggregated markets like eastern Washington State and northern Idaho. There are also Beacon Communities in large and midsized cities, including San Diego, Indianapolis, Detroit, Tulsa, and Cincinnati. It's really a diverse group with a diverse set of strategies.

Each Beacon Community has a portfolio of a dozen or so health IT projects, all trying to meet the triple aim of better health care, better health, and reduced cost.

The projects sort into three categories. First, build and strengthen health IT infrastructure and exchange capabilities. Second, improve cost, quality, and population health. Third, test innovative approaches to performance measurement, technology integration, and care delivery.

The Beacon Communities are healthcare markets that have already made important strides in health IT. The program is not about the federal government imposing a vision from outside, but about finding places where the addition of federal funds can be a difference maker both within those regional healthcare markets and across the country, as we help identify, develop, and spread best practices.

For example, one of the hotbeds for health IT going back over 30 years is Indianapolis, and specifically the Regenstrief Institute at Indiana University School of Medicine. Well known in Indiana, Sam Regenstrief (1909–1988) was one of America's least known but most successful entrepreneurs, the front-loading dishwasher king. He left the bulk of his fortune to medical research, and in the early 1980s the Regenstrief Institute was already envisioning the potential of electronic medical records. From this work, the community of Indianapolis helped lead the way in the electronic exchange of health information across the region through the Indiana Health Information Exchange.

The bottom line is that $12 million to $16 million over three years is a lot of money, but it's not a lot of money given the scope of the problems the Beacon Communities are trying to address. That is why we chose healthcare markets where there was already significant local investment and where competing health plans, hospitals, and physician groups were already coming together and establishing areas of collaboration in data sharing and analytics.

Here is a snapshot of the sorts of projects that Beacon Communities are doing in the first category I mentioned, building and strengthening health IT infrastructure and exchange capabilities.

One area in which several Beacon Communities are experimenting is remote patient monitoring. The concept makes perfect sense. But the literature is mixed. We don't know exactly why that is. And so Beacons are doing randomized trials on remote patient monitoring, for example.

Several of the Beacon Communities are deploying novel applications of the Direct Project, a simple, secure, scalable, standard-based way for participants to send authenticated, encrypted health information directly to known, trusted recipients over the Internet.

Sometimes the effort to build and strengthen means expanding something that is already working well. Indianapolis's Quality Health First program aggregates payer and clinical data and produces consistent performance measures that providers use to improve and health plans use to reward through Beacon that went from eight counties to statewide.

The second category of projects is improvement with regard to cost, quality, and population health. An important aspect of these and other Beacon Community projects is that they are required to produce performance measures, and they are accordingly making some very astute investments in structured measurement. This is producing great learning that ONC can share across the country.

For example, in Cincinnati, 30-day hospital readmission rates have turned in the right direction. And at the Keystone Beacon in central Pennsylvania, Geisinger is significantly lowering all-cause 30-day hospital readmission rates for patients with chronic heart or pulmonary problems.

That brings me to the third category of Beacon projects, innovation in performance measurement, technology integration, and care delivery.

Through a Beacon program in San Diego, EMTs are wirelessly transmitting 12-lead EKG data and other patient data from the field to hospital emergency rooms. Why is that important? You want the hospital cardiac team ready for when the EMTs roll you in with a heart attack. At the same time, hospitals don't want to prep resources and personnel for a heart attack that isn't really a heart attack. It costs about $10,000–$15,000 to get the cardiac catheterization lab and its team ready to treat a patient. In the first six months of this Beacon program, there's been a significant decrease in false positive activation of cardiac cath labs.

It also has improved right care when someone is having a heart attack, because the team at the hospital has advance information on the patient while EMS is rushing to them. So the team can start taking appropriate action as soon as the patient arrives. Recently a retired Navy admiral had a heart event as he was about to board an airplane in San Diego. Because the EMTs on the scene were able to send his data wirelessly to the hospital, he received exactly the treatment he needed as soon as he got to the hospital. He's now a huge spokesman for this particular project.

Cincinnati provides another good example of the power of health information exchange. Most private care doctors don't know when their patients show up in a hospital's emergency department. That's a problem. And so what do they do in

Cincinnati now? Irrespective of which hospital physicians are affiliated with, they receive a notification if any of their patients hit any emergency department in the region. And the physicians get this data in real time. So a medical assistant in a physician's office can look those up every day and contact the patients. It's a very simple intervention, but it has a profound effect on patients. They're saying, "Wow, I'm really impressed that you even knew I was in the hospital yesterday."

The Detroit and New Orleans Beacon Communities have co-designed a text messaging tool with Voxiva, a mobile health firm. This intervention reaches out to pre-diabetics and screens them for diabetes and then connects them to local resources. The tool knows your zip code and tells you, "Hey, there's a new diabetes clinic down the street that has resources for you," so it's very localized.

The Beacon Communities are proving to be great partners for ONC in increasing Meaningful Use of health IT and helping the country learn about what works. Ultimately we're all working together towards a technology infrastructure that supports accountable care. We're moving from independent kind of small mom-and-pop healthcare shops to integrated accountable systems. And maybe we're about halfway in between that path.

For example, the Beacon Community in Bangor, Maine, used the Beacon ONC funding to establish infrastructure for what is now the Bangor Beacon ACO, one of the CMS Innovation Center's 32 more advanced Pioneer ACOs. There are also Pioneer ACOs in the Beacon Communities in Detroit and Indianapolis that are highly leveraging the information exchange architecture regionally.

Three of the CMS Innovation Center's seven Comprehensive Primary Care Initiative sites are Beacon Communities. Working together with private sector health plans, CMS is testing new ways of financing primary care in the form of patient-centered medical homes.

It should be no surprise that these three regions were selected by CMS because the Beacon Communities have invested in technology, and they've invested in collaborative thinking about how to improve care in their market.

There are large challenges to progress in health IT. One of the most significant issues is that many private sector healthcare entities are not eager to participate in data sharing. They see their own data as a competitive asset, and their inclination is to hoard that data.

A related issue is that even when healthcare entities are willing to share data, their systems may not be interoperable. More generally, the more highly customized a data management system is, the less interoperability it has.

These two related issues of data hoarding and interoperability are especially problematic in terms of linking clinical data with payer data. We need to make these links so that patients' data can follow them seamlessly as they move from provider to provider within the same region or from one part of the country to another.

But the promise of health IT and the exchange of data are now being achieved in a remarkable way, in Beacon Communities and many other regions of the country.

Not too far down the road, we can envision a health IT infrastructure that transforms many areas of clinical and translational research. For example, large randomized trials of medical procedures and pharmaceuticals cost tens of millions of dollars to conduct in the USA. With privacy-protected data on sufficient numbers of patients, researchers could conduct virtual randomized trials at the cost of doing a database spread sheet that correlates the delivery of different procedures or medications with patient outcomes.

In short, this is really a great time when health IT and payment reform are quite visibly coming together in a synergistic way. From a federal perspective healthcare reform is a two-act play, where the first act is to "wire" the system and the second is to rethink the way we pay for care. The ACA is giving added impetus to these efforts and to the partnership between ONC and CMS.

Investments to promote the development and implementation of health IT provide needed momentum to change the way providers, health systems, and communities use healthcare data. Health information technology provides the infrastructure for providers and health systems to better manage the health of the populations they serve with the promise of delivering higher quality care at lower costs. While the health and quality benefits of IT-enabled interventions may be intuitive, it is less clear how these efforts are sustainable within a fee-for-service context where reducing hospitalizations and other health services reduces revenues.

It is here that the intersection of technology and payment policy is essential to transform the healthcare system. Payment reform creates a new business context for health IT. Due in part to the two-step passage of HITECH and the ACA, the synergy of health HIT implementation and payment reform is currently on display in dynamic fashion.

Chapter 9
Results from a Massachusetts Pilot Study

JudyAnn Bigby

My colleagues and I in the Commonwealth of Massachusetts Executive Office of Health and Human Services frequently receive requests from elsewhere in the country for help in refuting myths about healthcare reform. If the Affordable Care Act (ACA) is a national experiment in healthcare reform, then the healthcare reform law adopted in Massachusetts in 2006 and known as Chapter 58 is a virtual pilot study for it.[1] The Massachusetts law and the federal law have much in common, and they have been attacked by their opponents in much the same way. The upshot is that if the facts refute the opponents of healthcare reform in Massachusetts, they will likely do the same in regard to the ACA's national reforms.

The most common myths about healthcare reform in Massachusetts are:

- Massachusetts is proposing to ration health care to deal with the runaway cost of its healthcare reform.
- Massachusetts healthcare reform is highly unpopular with the public, the business community, and policy makers.
- The Massachusetts law is bankrupting the state.
- Significant numbers of Massachusetts residents are ignoring the mandate and only purchasing insurance when they need care.
- Massachusetts residents have higher premiums in the non-group market as a result of the healthcare reform law.
- The Massachusetts healthcare reform law is eroding employer-provided health insurance.
- The Massachusetts law has not significantly reduced the ranks of the uninsured in the state.

---

[1] Bills that become law during a session of the Massachusetts legislature are given "chapter" numbers based on the chronological order in which they were enacted. Chapter 58 of the Acts of 2006 is "An Act Providing Access to Affordable, Quality, Accountable Health Care."

J. Bigby, MD (✉)
Formerly Health and Human Services, State of Massachusetts, Boston, MA, USA
e-mail: Judyann.bigby@state.ma.us

H.P. Selker and J.S. Wasser (eds.), *The Affordable Care Act as a National Experiment:*
Health Policy Innovations and Lessons, DOI 10.1007/978-1-4614-8351-9_9,
© Springer Science+Business Media New York 2014

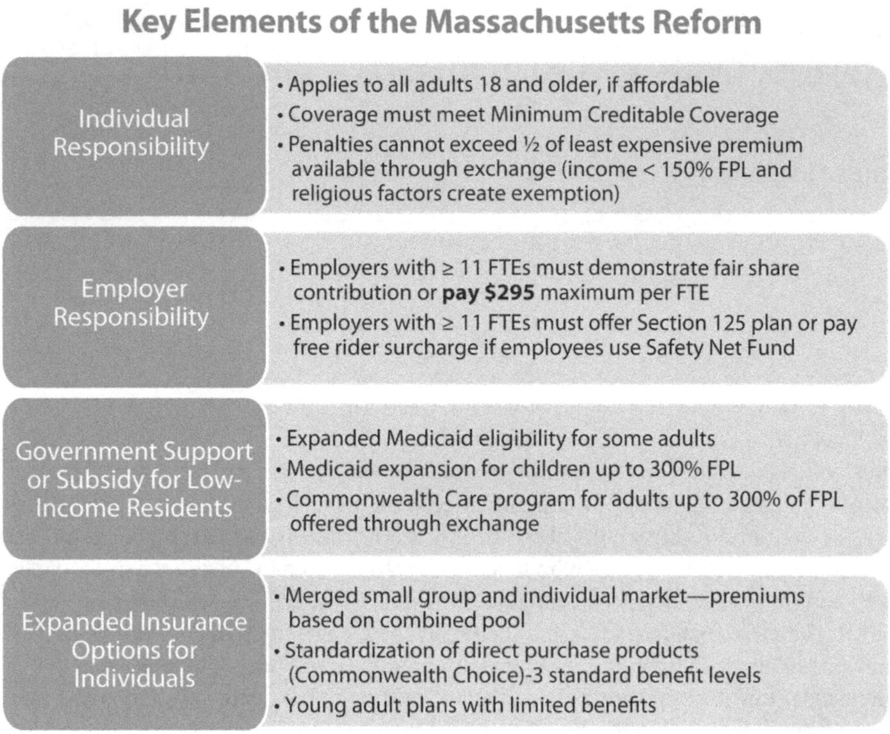

Key Elements of the Massachusetts Reform

Individual Responsibility	• Applies to all adults 18 and older, if affordable • Coverage must meet Minimum Creditable Coverage • Penalties cannot exceed ½ of least expensive premium available through exchange (income < 150% FPL and religious factors create exemption)
Employer Responsibility	• Employers with ≥ 11 FTEs must demonstrate fair share contribution or **pay $295** maximum per FTE • Employers with ≥ 11 FTEs must offer Section 125 plan or pay free rider surcharge if employees use Safety Net Fund
Government Support or Subsidy for Low-Income Residents	• Expanded Medicaid eligibility for some adults • Medicaid expansion for children up to 300% FPL • Commonwealth Care program for adults up to 300% of FPL offered through exchange
Expanded Insurance Options for Individuals	• Merged small group and individual market—premiums based on combined pool • Standardization of direct purchase products (Commonwealth Choice)-3 standard benefit levels • Young adult plans with limited benefits

Fig. 9.1 Key elements of the Massachusetts reform

• Healthcare reform in Massachusetts busted the primary care system and exacerbated a shortage of primary care doctors.

These assertions are all false. The facts show a different and very positive picture. Let's first look at the components of Chapter 58. Its key elements are also the foundation of federal healthcare reform via the ACA (Fig. 9.1).

The most important element of Chapter 58 is an individual responsibility to buy health insurance that applies to all adults, with the caveat that they have to have access to affordable insurance. If you're going to require people to buy health insurance, that insurance should actually provide adequate healthcare coverage, and thus the law also has a Minimum Creditable Coverage criterion.

The penalties for failing to buy health insurance cannot exceed half of the least expensive premium available through the health insurance exchange that the law established. People with incomes below 100 % of the federal poverty level and people with certain religious beliefs are exempted.

The employer responsibility required that any employer with 11 or more full-time equivalent (FTE) employees must make a fair share contribution to the employees' health insurance or pay $295 per FTE per year. The initial definition of fair share for a Massachusetts employer with 11–49 employees was that the employer contributes at least 33 % of the premium or demonstrates that at least 50 % of the employees take the employer's offer of health insurance. Employers with 50 or more FTE employees must contribute at least 33 % of their employees' health insurance premiums and 50 % take up the employer's offer of insurance, or they must demonstrate that at least 75 % of their FTE employees take up the offer of insurance regardless of what percent of the premium the employer offers to pay. (In August of 2012 the legislature revised the fair share definition to apply to employers with 21 or more FTE employees and allow employers to count as "covered" employees those that have insurance through a spouse or some other mechanism such as Medicare.) If employers of 11 or more FTEs don't sponsor their own insurance plan, they must offer a Section 125 cafeteria plan, which enables employees to use pretax dollars to pay health insurance premiums. Employers of 11 or more FTEs who don't sponsor their own insurance plan or offer a Section 125 cafeteria plan were required to pay a free rider surcharge if their employees use the Massachusetts Health Safety Net, a program for low-income residents or residents of any income whose medical costs exceed their means. A central feature of the Massachusetts healthcare reform is its expansion of coverage for low-income residents through government subsidies, including MassHealth, the Massachusetts Medicaid program, and the federal government-sponsored State Children's Health Insurance Plan (SCHIP). Using the 1115 Medicaid waiver authority, income eligibility expanded for some adults and most children up to incomes of 300 % of the federal poverty level. Whenever our waiver has come up for renewal, we have stressed the importance of maintaining eligibility up to 300 % of the federal poverty level especially for children.

The Commonwealth Care Program, which Chapter 58 established to offer free or subsidized health insurance for low-income residents, is also available to adults with incomes up to 300 % of the federal poverty level. Individuals pay premiums and co-pays in this program according to a sliding scale depending on their income. The state subsidizes the premiums and co-pays. Commonwealth Care products are one group of insurance products that are offered by the insurance exchange, the Health Connector.

Under Chapter 58 the state revised its long-standing uncompensated care program which paid hospitals and community health centers for uncompensated care and bad debt. The transformed program, the Health Safety Net, covers the cost of care provided by hospitals or community health centers to uninsured or underinsured individuals with incomes up to 400 % of the federal poverty level. The total amount of spending from the Health Safety Net is capped annually.

Chapter 58 increased access to affordable insurance for individuals above 300 % of the federal poverty level by creating the Health Connector, an independent state agency that helps Massachusetts residents find health insurance coverage and avoid tax penalties for being uninsured. The Connector provides an interface for individuals and small businesses to identify Commonwealth Choice insurance products in the merged individual and small group market that are affordable and comprehensive. Merging the private insurance small group and individual markets was designed to bring down premiums for individuals. The price for individuals decreased significantly while small business premiums slightly increased.

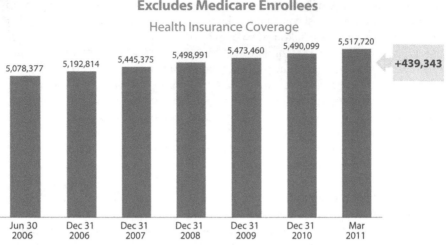

Fig. 9.2 The number of individuals enrolled in health insurance plans in Massachusetts increased steadily over a 5 year period (Sources: Membership reported to Massachusetts Division of Health Care Finance and Policy by health plans, and Mass Health; Commonwealth care enrollment data are from the Health Connector)

The Connector worked with private insurers to create a range of products for individuals who purchase insurance from among the Commonwealth Choice plans on the exchange. The Connector standardized these products and ranked them as bronze, silver, or gold medal plans, so that purchasers could easily understand what they were buying and how it compared to other plans. There are three tiers of benefits—low, medium, and high—in bronze medal plans and two tiers of benefits—low and high—in silver medal plans.

Massachusetts also created young adult plans for people aged 18–26. These plans have slightly fewer benefits than other plans. Chapter 58 also allowed adult children to stay on their parents' insurance until they were 26 or up to 2 years after they were not claimed as a dependent.

Those are the foundation elements of Chapter 58, and they are also foundation elements of the ACA. Now let's look at the results in Massachusetts as a preview of what the results of the ACA may be, beginning with the number of Massachusetts residents, excluding Medicare enrollees, who have health insurance (Fig. 9.2).

The June 2006 bar in Fig. 9.2 shows the number of Massachusetts residents with health insurance just after Chapter 58 was passed by the legislature and signed by the governor in Spring 2006. By October the Commonwealth Health Connector was up and running, and the December 2006 bar already shows a substantial increase in the number of people covered. As of March 2011, we estimated that 439,000 more people had acquired health insurance compared to before reform. Counting Medicare enrollees, Massachusetts had thus reached the point of near-universal coverage for its approximately 6.5 million residents. Another way of looking at this is to calculate the Massachusetts uninsurance rate (Fig. 9.3).

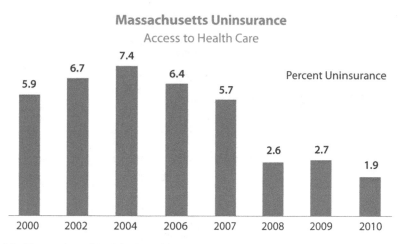

Fig. 9.3 The number of individuals without health insurance declined over a 5-year period in Massachusetts (Sources: Massachusetts Division of Health Care Finance and Policy Household Surveys for 2000, 2002, 2004, 2006, and 2007; surveys from 2000 through 2006 were conducted February through June of the survey year; survey for 2007 was conducted January through July of 2007. Data for 2008, 2009 and 2010 are from the Urban Institute tabulation on the Massachusetts Health Insurance Survey for the respective years. For more information, visit www.mass.gov/dhcfp. Click on the "Publication and Analyses", then go to "Household Health Insurance Survey." National uninsured rate is as reported by the US Census Bureau in Income, Poverty, and Health Insurance Coverage in the United States, 2008 and 2009 data. http://www.census.gov.)

The Massachusetts uninsurance rate has decreased from 6.4 % at the time of reform to 1.9 % in 2010. Opponents of healthcare reform have criticized this number because it is not consistent with the uninsurance rate in the US Census Bureau data. The percentages in Fig. 9.3 come from an annual survey of households, conducted by the Urban Institute for the Massachusetts Division of Health Care Finance and Policy, that is specifically designed to capture uninsurance rates, which is not the main aim of the Census Bureau's household surveys. Differences in the estimates of the rate of uninsurance from the surveys reflect many factors, including differences in the wording of the insurance questions asked in the surveys, differences in question placement and context, and differences in survey design and fielding strategies, among other things. At about 4 % and 1.9 %, respectively, the US Census Bureau and Massachusetts estimates of the uninsurance rate in the state are not that far apart. More significant, surely, is that the Census Bureau estimates the uninsurance rate nationally to be about 16 %.

As envisioned by Chapter 58, the growth in the insured population in Massachusetts has come primarily from people with incomes at or near the federal poverty level (Fig. 9.4).

About two-thirds of the people who have gained health insurance since reform began have incomes at 150 % of the federal poverty level or below. This underscores how important it is to have subsidies for the low-income populations. MassHealth enrollment has grown by about 300,000 people from 2006 to 2011. And the number

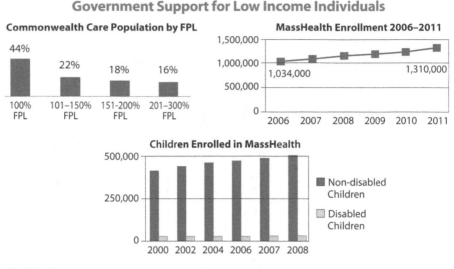

Fig. 9.4 Government support helped enroll low-income adults and children

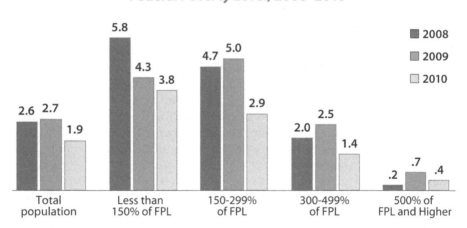

Fig. 9.5 Percent of uninsured Massachusetts residents by federal poverty level, 2008–2010 (Source: Urban Institute tabulations on the 2008, 2009, and 2010 Massachusetts Health Insurance Survey for the Massachusetts Division of Health Care Finance and Policy. For more information, visit www.mass.gov/dhcfp. Click on "Publications and Analyses", then go to "Household Health Insurance Survey.")

of children covered by Massachusetts CHIP has grown from 410,000 in 2006 to about 512,000 in 2011. Examining the uninsurance rates by income level in a little more detail offers additional evidence of the need for subsidized health insurance for the low-income populations. It also reveals the success of Chapter 58 in meeting that need (Fig. 9.5).

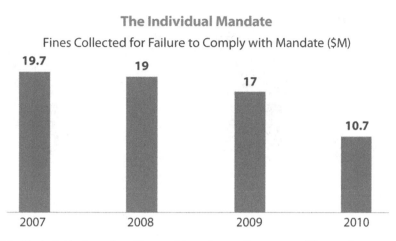

The Individual Mandate

Fines Collected for Failure to Comply with Mandate ($M)

19.7	19	17	10.7
2007	2008	2009	2010

Fig. 9.6 The individual mandate. (Source: Massachusetts Department of Revenue)

For the total population of Massachusetts, the rate of uninsurance was already fairly low in 2008 and 2009, but it decreased quite a bit in 2010. There were significant decreases in uninsurance, from much higher starting points, for people with incomes less than 150 % and 300 % of the federal poverty level. The decrease in uninsurance for people with incomes from 300 % to 499 % of the federal income level roughly matched the decrease in uninsurance for the total population. And as one might expect, there was only a slight decrease in uninsurance, from a much lower starting point, for people with incomes that were 500 % of the federal poverty level or higher.

Both Chapter 58 and the ACA include a penalty for those individuals who fail to comply with the mandate to buy health insurance. Revenue from collection of the Chapter 58 penalty provides another gauge of the law's success in reducing uninsurance in Massachusetts. In 2007 collections were $19.7 million, and in 2010 they were $10.7 million. I suspect that the final tally of 2011 collections will probably slightly increase over 2010 because of the continuing impact of the recession (Fig. 9.6).

What about access? One of the myths I mentioned was that healthcare reform in Massachusetts busted the primary care system and exacerbated a shortage of primary care doctors. Yet an annual survey we do of the impact of reform reveals a reality at odds with the myth (Fig. 9.7).

Since reform more people report having a usual source of care outside of the emergency department. This would not be possible if it were true that healthcare reform broke the limits of the primary care system and the availability of primary care doctors in Massachusetts. The facts also reveal that the biggest percentage increases in access to a usual care provider outside the emergency department occurred among low-income residents. This represents additional proof that Chapter 58 is accomplishing its goals of extending health insurance coverage to disadvantaged population groups, while also helping to constrain healthcare cost growth.

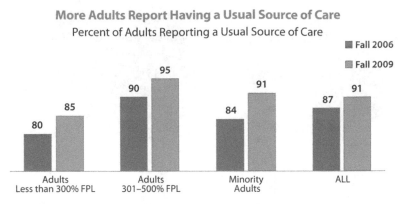

Fig. 9.7 After a 3-year period, more Massachusetts adults had an identified source of medical care (Source: Massachusetts Health Reform Survey 2010)

It is extremely expensive to provide basic medical care through emergency departments, and reducing the basic medical care burden on emergency departments is accordingly an important goal of both Chapter 58 and the ACA.

The impact of Chapter 58 to improve access to care for disadvantaged populations was described in a study by Pande et al. published in the *American Journal of Preventive Medicine*. They found that living in Massachusetts in 2009 was associated with a higher probability of being insured, a lower probability of foregoing care because of cost, and a higher probability of having a personal doctor, compared to expected levels in the absence of reform, defined by trends in control states and adjusting for socioeconomic factors.

One of the reasons people gained access to care outside the emergency department was that Chapter 58 supported more people's access to the 54 community health centers in Massachusetts. In the first year after reform was enacted, the health centers added more than 70,000 people to their rolls, and they have seen continued enrollment growth since 2007. The community health centers were proactive in preparing for the influx of newly insured individuals through MassHealth and Commonwealth Care. The fact that Massachusetts has such a vigorous community health center system has served the state well. The ACA envisions similar use of community health centers, rather than hospital emergency departments, across the country (Fig. 9.8).

What happened to employer-sponsored health insurance because of Chapter 58? Unfortunately for those who wanted us to fail, employers did not stop offering health insurance (Fig. 9.9).

In fact, the offer rate went up in Massachusetts, with the percentage of employers offering insurance rising from 70 % in 2005, the year before reform, to 77 % in 2010. The national rate in 2010 was about 69 %, compared to 60 % in 2005. However, Massachusetts experienced a decline in the percent of premium costs covered by employers from 2006 to 2010. But this same trend also occurred in the rest of the country, and it cannot be attributed to Chapter 58.

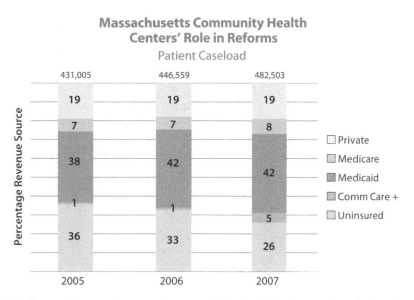

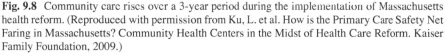

Fig. 9.8 Community care rises over a 3-year period during the implementation of Massachusetts health reform. (Reproduced with permission from Ku, L. et al. How is the Primary Care Safety Net Faring in Massachusetts? Community Health Centers in the Midst of Health Care Reform. Kaiser Family Foundation, 2009.)

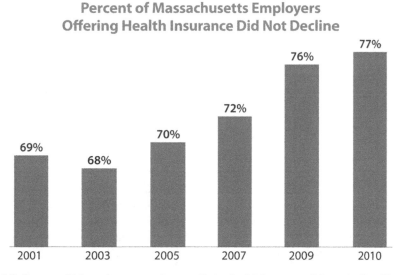

Fig. 9.9 Percent of Massachusetts employers offering health insurance did not decline (Sources: Massachusetts Division of Health Care Finance and Policy Employer surveys for selected years in the period 2001-2010. For further information on the DHCFP Employer Survey Report, visit www. mass.gov/dhcfp and follow the "Publication and Analyses" link.)

Fig. 9.10 Fair share
contribution. Source:
Massachusetts Division of
Health Care Finance and
Policy

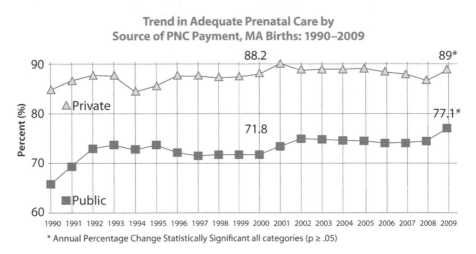

Fair Share Contribution

• 95% of employers subject to the Fair Share requirement meet the standard for a reasonable contribution

• 4.6% were liable for the fair share assessment

• Lowest levels of compliance was among restaurants, and temp agencies

• Over the first 4 years of the law assessments average about $15M per year

Trend in Adequate Prenatal Care by Source of PNC Payment, MA Births: 1990–2009

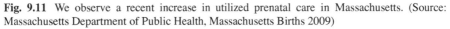

* Annual Percentage Change Statistically Significant all categories (p ≥ .05)

Fig. 9.11 We observe a recent increase in utilized prenatal care in Massachusetts. (Source: Massachusetts Department of Public Health, Massachusetts Births 2009)

Let's examine other impacts on employers. Among the 95 % of employers that are subject to the fair share contribution because they have 11 or more FTE employees, only 4.6 % have been found to be liable for the assessment. The lowest levels of employer compliance with the fair share contribution requirement are in the restaurant industry and temporary worker agencies. From 2007 to 2010 the total assessments on employers who did not make fair share contributions averaged about $15 million per year. So the sky has not fallen for employers as a result of Chapter 58 (Fig. 9.10).

The numbers we've looked at so far don't capture the entirety of the human dimension of Chapter 58. If we want to understand the difference it makes when people gain access to care, we need to look at health outcomes, things such as the rate at which pregnant women receive adequate prenatal care (Fig. 9.11).

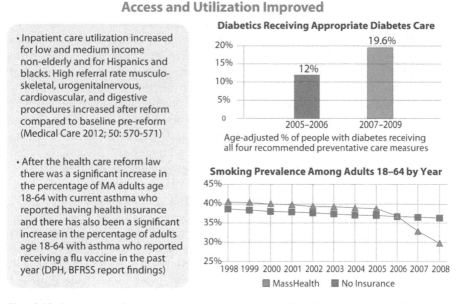

Fig. 9.12 In the last few years, several important health indicators improve throughout Massachusetts

Before Chapter 58, the lines are relatively flat for the percentages of women with either public or private health insurance who received adequate prenatal care.

After Chapter 58, however, and for the first time since we've been tracking this data, going back to 1991, we actually see an indication that more women are getting adequate prenatal care. If you think about it, it makes sense that if you give more people access to continuous health coverage, when women get pregnant, they're already in the system and will get care. This is obviously something that we will continue to study as we track the impact of Chapter 58 and related follow-on legislation over time.

We also have other highly positive data on how care access and utilization have improved since Chapter 58 became law (Fig. 9.12).

The top left corner of Fig. 9.12 refers to a 2012 article in *Medical Care* showing that inpatient care utilization in five different categories of procedures — musculoskeletal, urogenital, nervous, cardiovascular, and digestive — increased among low- and medium-income non-elderly residents and among Hispanics and Blacks after reform. The study did not assess the appropriateness of care in these instances. But given what we know about population group health disparities and underutilization in the five care categories, the increases are almost certainly good news.

The lower left and upper right corners of Fig. 9.12 likewise refer to the Massachusetts Department of Public Health (DPH) findings of improvements in care access and utilization for people with asthma and diabetes since reform.

Compared to the 2005–2006 period, more people with asthma reported having insurance in the 2009–2010 period, and during that same period, the percent of asthmatics who reported receiving a flu shot increased from 36 % to 48 %. We have also seen an increase, from 12.7 % in 2005–2006 to 19.6 % in 2007–2009, in the number of diabetics who received appropriate care (annual eye exam, annual foot exam for numbness, flu shot, and twice yearly A1c check).

The lower right corner of Fig. 9.12 shows how smoking prevalence has changed since Chapter 58 required coverage for smoking cessation treatment in the MassHealth program. There has been a more than 10 % decrease in smoking among the MassHealth-covered population. We also found there was a decline in emergency department visits for asthma, chronic obstructive pulmonary disease (COPD), and acute chest pain, all of which are strongly associated with smoking. This also translated into significant financial savings in the MassHealth program.

Did reform bust the Massachusetts budget? Our own analysis and third-party analysis both indicate that state budget spending on health reform amounted to less than 1 % of the total state spending in the budget. This is a very hard thing to analyze because we did reform and then the recession hit. It is also true that overall spending on healthcare reform has been shared. The Blue Cross Foundation found that individuals, government, and employers have all increased spending on health insurance at a rate proportional to their spending prior to reform.

However, one of the reasons we know that our health reform strategy works is that during the recession, when our unemployment rate went up to close to 9 %, the number of uninsured did not increase in the state. The state was able to pay for the increased enrollment in government-subsidized programs due to enhanced federal funding for Medicaid under President Obama's stimulus bill, the American Recovery and Reinvestment Act of 2009.

Affordability of health care is a big issue in Massachusetts, as it is in the rest of the country. Affordability really goes hand in hand with an individual mandate to buy insurance (Fig. 9.13).

Figure 9.13 shows individual, employer, and government contributions to health insurance premiums in 2008 for both private and public plans. The first bar on the left shows the premium for an individual covered by the Massachusetts Group Insurance Commission (GIC), which provides health insurance to Massachusetts state employees, retirees, and their dependents. The second bar shows the mean premium payment for employer-based plans. Bars three to six show the premiums and the extent of government subsidy—calculated based on income in relation to the federal poverty level—for health insurance under Commonwealth Care. The remaining bars show the premiums for Commonwealth Choice plans. The horizontal lines benchmark the maximum affordable premiums according to the affordability standard determined by the Health Connector for people with incomes of $37,500, $42,500, and $52,500. People with incomes below $37,500 generally qualified for subsidized coverage under Commonwealth Care. The dollar figures are a little bit out of date, but the proportional contributions would be much the same with more recent premium data.

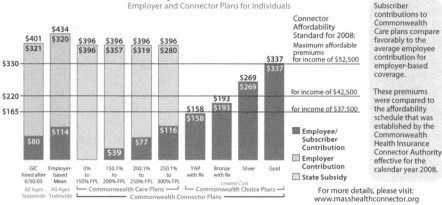

Fig. 9.13 A variety of health plans and premiums are offered by the Commonwealth, including those targeted to low-income individuals. (Source: Massachusetts Division of Health Care Finance and Policy)

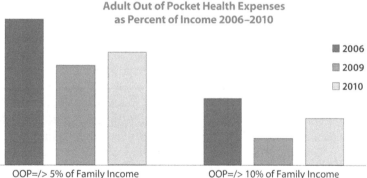

Fig. 9.14 Out-of-pocket medical expenses decline with Massachusetts health reform (Source: Massachusetts Division of Health Care Finance and Policy Massachusetts Health Reform Survey)

In surveying individual consumers, we have asked them about changes in their out-of-pocket health expenses as a percentage of their income (Fig. 9.14).

Initially the percentage of people who said that out-of-pocket medical expenses represented more than 5 % or 10 % of their family income declined after reform. Rates started to go up again in 2010, likely because of the continuing impact of the recession, and this is very concerning to us. But the percentage remains significantly below what it was before Chapter 58.

One of the reasons why the Massachusetts experiment in healthcare reform has been so successful is that the state invested about $3 million a year for several years to make sure that there was outreach to find people who did not have health insurance. This created a lot of confusion in 2007 and early 2008 because of the rapidity with which people were identified and signed up for state-subsidized health insurance. The rapidity with which people were being enrolled in Commonwealth Care suggested that the uninsurance rate in Massachusetts had to be much higher than estimated. But this turned out not to be so. The initial rise in enrollment was so great because the outreach was extremely effective. Enrollment in the Commonwealth Care program has remained steady at about 160,000 people for several years now.

Overall spending for uncompensated care in Massachusetts decreased by 40 %. However, it is important to keep in mind that neither Massachusetts nor federal healthcare reform covers undocumented people. Those people still need care.

One thing that surprised us was the extent to which people were jumping in and out of insurance coverage based on their perceived healthcare needs. They were signing up for coverage just before they anticipated needing significant care and dropping it afterwards. Although the percentage of total premiums affected by this behavior was not huge—they were less than 0.1 % of total premiums at most—it was still significant enough that we had to implement a fixed enrollment period so that people wouldn't get and then discard health insurance after they had an elective procedure or some other temporary need for treatment. This is an example of the kind of follow-on adjustment that successful healthcare reform required. In reflecting on Chapter 58, we have to remember that healthcare reform in Massachusetts did not start in 2006. It began at least as far back as 1988, when then-Governor Dukakis signed a comprehensive reform bill. Although much of the bill was later repealed, certain provisions such as consumer protections to prevent denial of insurance coverage, access to Medicaid-funded independent living and community supports for the disabled, and coverage for disabled working adults were maintained and were an important foundation for ongoing reforms. Chapter 58 addressed policies that contributed to the uninsured rate in Massachusetts and proposed ways to fill in the gaps. Through the recession we had the opportunity to test whether the model worked, and as people lost their employer-sponsored insurance, they were able to come onto the MassHealth and Commonwealth Care insurance rolls. The programs were in place to help people when they needed it most.

To return to the view of Chapter 58 as a pilot program for the ACA, I think the most powerful understanding of the results of healthcare reform come from consumers. Shortly after Governor Deval Patrick appointed me as Secretary of Health and Human Services in Massachusetts, the owner of the dry cleaner I go to asked me if the health reform bill would do any good for him and his employees. None of them had had health insurance coverage for as long as they could remember.

They all signed up for insurance through the Health Connector. A few Saturdays later, the sister of the owner told me that she had gone for her first physical in 25 years, since the birth of her daughter. She said, "Now I know why my vision isn't so good. I have cataracts. Not only that, I'm going to get them fixed and I won't have to pay anything." That's the kind of story we hear again and again thanks to Chapter 58. In April 2012, Dr. Lynda Young, the immediate past president of the Massachusetts Medical Society, told me that she has not seen one uninsured child in her practice in five years. That is an incontrovertible marker of the success of fact-based, myth-busting healthcare reform in Massachusetts. It should be a harbinger of the benefits the whole country will experience from the ACA.

Part III
Make it a People Issue: Engaging the Public

Chapter 10
Commentary on Part III: Engaging the Public

June S. Wasser

"Healthy citizens are the greatest asset any country can have."[1]

Who can argue that a healthy citizenry is a necessary prerequisite for a thriving nation? And yet does it necessarily follow that the national government is responsible for individual, community, and public health? In short, liberals say yes, and conservatives say no.

How this controversy plays out on the national scene and its very important impact on legislative policy and on state and individual rights has been discussed throughout this volume. Section III in particular discusses how both the individual and society will benefit from understanding the ACA and its implementation. Society in this context includes healthcare systems, businesses, industry, and the public sphere of neighborhoods, local healthcare organizations, patients, etc.

And yet it would appear that the public, i.e., patients or consumers, are not always inclined to accept the ACA as a national benefit or public good. Public opinion polls in this section are discussed by Bruce Landon with Stuart Altman and again by Ceci Connolly. These polls illustrate that opinions change through time, depending on the extent and effectiveness of the messaging. Whereas in real estate it is "location, location, location" that matters, in politics and policy, it is "messaging, messaging, messaging...."

Connolly, in her following chapter, reports that the popularity of the ACA mirrored President Obama's popularity. Support of the ACA was highest immediately following his election to his first term in office and began to steadily fall through the end of summer 2009 when the ACA messaging battle was finally lost. Furthermore, while the public acknowledged even in 2009 that the ACA offered a public good in

[1] Churchill WS. The war speeches of Winston S. Churchill, OM, CH, PC, MP, Volume two: from June 25, 1941 to September 6, 1943. London: Cassell & Company Ltd; 1965.

J.S. Wasser, MS (✉)
Tufts University School of Medicine, Boston, MA, USA
e-mail: June.Wasser@tufts.edu

H.P. Selker and J.S. Wasser (eds.), *The Affordable Care Act as a National Experiment:*
Health Policy Innovations and Lessons, DOI 10.1007/978-1-4614-8351-9_10,
© Springer Science+Business Media New York 2014

terms of improving the overall healthcare of the nation by helping those most in need or the uninsured, on an individual level, when it came to helping patients and families, there was little recognition of a personal benefit.

Landon and Altman point out that as recently as November 2012 public opinion polls continued to show confusion and ambivalence. Similar polls reported by the media in the first half of 2013 echo the same results. In fact, the longer objective discussions of the ACA are absent from the daily news, the more skeptical the public becomes. So, what went wrong with the rollout and communications about the ACA?

Republican opposition to the legislation led to an early campaign of negative messaging. The threat of "death panels" easily comes to mind. The White House was so reluctant to take this threat seriously (thinking, nor could anyone else) that it did not respond. Strike one. The White House should have taken the lead position when it came to communicating about a new legislative plan they were proposing. Strike two was when they did not immediately respond to negative attack ads from their critics.

During the summer of 2009, there existed a great deal of uncertainty about the ACA even in the White House. DC insiders were acutely aware that the President was of yet uncertain about what he could comfortably support in the final piece of legislation. Without a full commitment and communication plan to follow suit, there was little opportunity to gain the popular support necessary for achieving a clear and quick win on the issue of national healthcare reform.

In the following pages, John McDonough lays out four stages necessary for healthcare reform. The first stage is access to care for the vast majority of the populace. The second stage is delivery system reform that includes improvements and innovation in information technology, patient safety, and quality of care. The third stage of healthcare reform focuses on wellness and prevention initiatives. The last stage is to embrace health issues in all policies affecting people whether it is a governmental policy originating in the Departments of Agriculture, Defense, Energy, Housing, etc. Coordination amongst all government departments and agencies would be the goal to strive for.

In the rollout of the ACA, stage I, or access to care, became the single most important message. After all, access to care and its financial savings (relieving the burden of critical care to the uninsured and underinsured) is the reason the legislation was produced, that is, to guarantee that all who are ill can afford care and that there would no longer be restrictions on medical preconditions or lack of prior insurance coverage or limitations for those up to 26 years of age and continuing on parental health plans. And yet Americans remain confused about any gains they may have made through the new law.

When national opinion polls indicate that ACA legislation will benefit a minority of the population and not the majority, there is a failure to consider the unpredictability of catastrophic illness or accidents. Equally unpredictable is the loss of insurance or the lack of affordable insurance in times of financial difficulty or job loss.

Who will provide a safety net from these burdens? Like Medicare, Medicaid, Social Security, and other social safety net programs, it is to the federal government that we look for relief. And yet Americans are confused about these gains. They are confused that we can spend additional federal dollars providing access to care and then save on dollars caring for critically ill populations not now completely covered.

It is confusing, and many of those who support the ACA do so because they have long and deep commitments to social programs, not because they can quote the legislation in detail. It requires more effort to reach people who otherwise are less supportive of social programs in general or, better yet, want to know what the government is doing to help them and their families. Outreach efforts, communications, and messaging can make the difference between support, apathy, and cynicism.

What confounds the situation we find ourselves in is that the Obama campaign apparatus is applauded for being the very best tactical operation of its kind. The grassroots outreach efforts, organization of people across the country, and extremely deliberate and strategic messaging won him not only the 2008 election but the 2012 reelection in a time of dire financial uncertainty. This is a President with an operation that knows how to win. And yet it can be argued that the commitment to winning the communications battle over this very important piece of healthcare legislation was lacking.

Let us consider the other major changes ACA will usher in beyond "simple" access. Imagine we now live in a world where every American has health insurance and easy access to practitioners. Does that mean our care is better or more affordable? No, as McDonough points out, we still need to implement health system reform and preventive/wellness services.

There was effectively little to no messaging about the safety and quality of care in this country that stands to improve through ACA implementation. Medicine is a science and like all sciences is hypothesis driven. Its specialized knowledge expands almost daily, based on rigorous scientific research and evidence. Our healthcare system needs to respond accordingly. New medical technologies, the ever-expanding medical drug and device market, discoveries of new illnesses and treatment modalities, what works and what does not work when applied to patient or population health—these are all new and exciting avenues of exploration in a field as old as antiquity. Beyond access to care, the ACA proposes to vastly improve the quality of care so our population as a whole lives healthier and longer while at the same time decreases the costs of care—an even greater gain for our nation.

As discussed by Landon and Altman, there is no single value proposition for the public; rather, the ACA affects different people in different ways. This makes the legislation a much more complicated law to describe and requires multiple messages aimed at different audiences. That departs greatly from the singular message of access to care for all.

Landon and Altman point out that when assessing the value proposition of the ACA, it is the focus on preventive care that will positively affect population health and the public. Perhaps, if the communication's focus all along had been on preventive care and population health, then the public would have understood why individual access to care was a necessary precursor.

Another point long lost in the discussion of public engagement and support for the ACA is the probability that if little or no value is embraced by the public, those who stand to benefit most, those who are uninsured or without appropriate care, will not sign up for new insurance options provided by exchanges at the state and federal levels. This would not only be unfortunate for the populace but would doom the ACA to failure as the intended outcomes would not have been achieved. The strength of the legislation is in enrolling as many people as possible to achieve both economic and wellness efficiencies.

Ineffective outreach and communications resulted in underwhelming support by the public for national healthcare reform. The final piece of legislation can be argued as a much watered-down version of a grand plan to make us competitive with our international counterparts on critical medical measures like mortality and safety and cost. Strike three in this communications battle for reform was not deliberately engaging the public in a meaningful way. Without an actual understanding of the law and its proposed personal and community benefits, there was little embracing of these tenets and certainly no leadership on behalf of the public to demand that they receive what is their due—quality of care at lower costs.

Strike three and you are out; so was the battle lost? In this volume we celebrate the passage of the ACA and the great win on the part of the Obama administration for their efforts and hard work. There is no doubt it will be one, if not the greatest, of the President's legacies. And as with many policies, this is only the first iteration aimed at healthcare reform. As the ACA evolves we will learn new lessons and make even greater strides to improve our policies and laws. Or so we hope.

Politics are unpredictable. The longest serving Justice in the history of the Supreme Court of the United States, Associate Justice William O. Douglas, in his famous opinion on free speech and the sale of pornographic journals (Dissenting, *Kingsley Books, Inc. v. Brown*, 354 U.S. 436, 447 (1957) is credited with saying, "The audience ... that hissed yesterday may applaud today, even for the same performance." Such is the court of public opinion.

It would seem that government in its righteous cause to provide for its citizens would engage those very same citizens in those very same causes. Campaigning does not end once a President sits in the Oval Office. Winning the Oval Office is just the beginning of a long-term relationship with the public that requires an intimate understanding of public opinion and the forces that influence opinion. At least it is so in a democracy.

Peter Baker reported in a personal interview that was published in an October 12, 2010 New York Times article, "Education of a President"—closely preceding the midterm elections on these very lessons, Barack Obama affirmed, "...And I think anybody who has occupied this office has to remember that success is determined by an intersection in policy and politics and that you can't be neglecting of marketing and PR and public opinion."

Immediately following President Obama's historic reelection to a second term in office, his campaign turned to promoting policy. The reelection campaign organization, Obama for America, changed its name and operations to Organizing for Action. The new group is being led by his previous campaign advisors with input from his top political aides. The agenda is to now push legislation rather than politics. Clearly, there is recognition in the White House of lessons learned.

Chapter 11
The Value Proposition for Individuals and the Public

Bruce E. Landon and Stuart Altman

Introduction

The Patient Protection and Affordable Care Act (ACA) of 2010 represents the single most important piece of healthcare legislation since the passage of Medicare and Medicaid in 1965. When fully implemented, the law will extend insurance coverage to approximately 25 million Americans who had previously lacked insurance while also reforming the market for individual and small group insurance [1, 2]. Those who are unable to obtain health insurance through their employers will now have reliable options for obtaining insurance on their own. As important, for the first time, the law puts almost all citizens on the same playing field with a collective responsibility for helping to reduce the cost of healthcare services.

Yet, despite these enormous accomplishments and the many benefits the bill provides, the Act remains deeply unpopular. Even with the recent reelection of President Obama to a second term, polling shows that only 43 % of the population supports the bill and fully 33 % want to repeal it in full [3]. Moreover, in health tracking polls, 53 % admit to being "confused" about the law [4]. That the law is unpopular and poorly understood should not come as a surprise; many of its key features have been misrepresented in the recent election and there is a general lack of understanding of the main features of the reform and what this will entail. The ACA should be considered a monumental accomplishment, but for it to live up to this potential, the general public needs a greater understanding of what the law does—and does not—set to accomplish.

B.E. Landon, MD, MBA, MSC (✉)
Department of Health Care Policy, Harvard Medical School, Boston, MA, USA
e-mail: landon@hcp.med.harvard.edu

S. Altman, PhD
The Heller School for Social Policy and Management, Brandeis University, Waltham, MA, USA
e-mail: altman@brandeis.edu

H.P. Selker and J.S. Wasser (eds.), *The Affordable Care Act as a National Experiment:* 91
Health Policy Innovations and Lessons, DOI 10.1007/978-1-4614-8351-9_11,
© Springer Science+Business Media New York 2014

The ACA is a complex law, running over 2,000 pages, and it will affect people in many different ways. Thus, there is no single "value proposition" that applies uniformly throughout the population. Rather, the value of the ACA differs for different populations. We believe, however, that the most important underlying aspects of the value of health reform lie in three principal areas. First, and most importantly, the ACA extends health insurance coverage to the majority of the uninsured by subsidizing the purchase of private insurance and expanding the eligibility for government-supported Medicaid benefits. Second, the ACA implements significant and important reforms of the individual and small group insurance markets and adds several provisions that will improve all forms of health insurance. Finally, the law establishes a number of changes in the way Medicare pays providers with the intent to significantly change the structure of the healthcare delivery system so as to lower healthcare costs. Below, we discuss each of these in more detail.

Assuring Coverage Is a Major Accomplishment

Quoting Harry Truman, Lyndon Johnson said on the signing of the legislation enacting Medicare and Medicaid, "Millions of our citizens do not now have a full measure of opportunity to achieve and to enjoy good health. Millions do not now have protection or security against the economic effects of sickness. And the time has now arrived for action to help them attain that opportunity and to help them get that protection." Prior to the passage of the ACA, there were 52 million uninsured Americans, with another 29 million being underinsured [5]. About three-quarters of the uninsured were members of working families. Even prior to the 2008 recession, the insurance coverage among adults was declining due to a steady decrease in employer-sponsored insurance. Thus, it is likely that over time, the uninsured rate would have become markedly higher and reached more into the middle class. Thus, absent passage of the ACA, it is likely that in the future, universal coverage could not have been accomplished within the broad structure of our current mixed private–public system. With only a deeply unpopular single-payer approach as an alternative, universal coverage within the USA may have been impossible.

Among the developed countries in the Organization for Economic Co-operation Development (OECD), the United States was the only country that lacked universal or near-universal coverage, yet healthcare spending per capita in the USA is more than twice the OECD average [6]. In addition, health outcomes and life expectancy trail the OECD average and the USA ranks second among OECD countries in the burden of chronic disease. Simply stated, despite excessive spending, the current system was not working well for large portions of the populations.

When fully implemented, the ACA will extend insurance coverage to an additional 25 million Americans, with just over half obtaining coverage under Medicaid (this number has been decreased somewhat because of the large number of states that chose not to participate in Medicaid expansion) and another 11.5 million through subsidized coverage through a state-run or federal-run health insurance exchange [7]. A relatively small residual (about 10 %) will need to purchase their own health insurance on the private markets, and the relatively few firms with more than 50 employees that don't already offer health insurance will be encouraged to do so by the threat of penalties for those who don't offer coverage. Thus, approximately 90 % of those obtaining coverage will be obtaining it through a federal program, and some portion of the residual includes young adults for whom the ACA requires coverage under their parents' policies and employees of small businesses who receive extensive tax credits to cover the cost of providing insurance coverage.

More impressively, the ACA extends insurance coverage without causing major disruptions to the healthcare system for those who have insurance coverage. Those who currently obtain their coverage from an employer will continue to do so with just small changes in their coverage that have few implications for costs (e.g., coverage of birth control at no cost was not common). In addition, those covered by Medicare or state Medicaid programs will also see little to no change, despite some reductions in the growth of payments to Medicare providers.

For the most part these reductions will be more than made up by increases in provider payments from the newly insured. Although large numbers of Americans lacked insurance coverage, this does not equate with them fully lacking access to healthcare services. For instance, under the Federal EMTALA (Emergency Medical Treatment and Active Labor Act) statute, emergency rooms are compelled to offer care to all and face strict penalties for failing to comply. Hospitals and physicians also continue to provide extensive medical services to patients without insurance. The costs of caring for the uninsured, however, are not free. Rather, much of these costs are borne by the insured who often are asked to pay more than necessary for their care to help pay for the care of those who lack coverage. The system has evolved to include an elaborate web of cross subsidization and pricing strategies that drive up premiums and generate unintended negative consequences. For instance, the inflated "list" price of hospital services are paid by very few consumers of care, but those without insurance coverage are often subject to these outlandishly high costs.

Despite these potential achievements, there also are some reasons to temper our enthusiasm. In June 2012, the Supreme Court ruled that individual states may choose to opt out of Medicaid expansion. According to data from the Kaiser Family Foundation, 21 states are not planning to expand Medicaid and another six continue to debate the issue. As written, the ACA precludes subsidies for those earning less then 100 % of the Federal Poverty Limit, so in these states the poorest populations who would have newly qualified for Medicaid generally will not be eligible for Federal subsidies to purchase insurance on the exchanges. Moreover, the states that have elected not to expand Medicaid include some of those with the largest numbers of poor uninsured and the least generous Medicaid programs. In addition, the Centers for Medicare and Medicaid services recently delayed the implementation until 2015 of the employer mandate, which requires employers with 50 or more full time equivalent employees to offer health insurance. Thus, recent estimates of the number of uninsured who will gain coverage under the ACA have been decreased by approximately 5 million people nationally (from over 30 million to approximately 25 million). Finally, there also is growing concern that the federal exchange may not be able to handle the extra burden of the large number of states that elected not to operate their own exchanges [8].

Health Insurance Market Reforms Will Be a Boon to Many

Although expansion of eligibility for Medicaid and the subsidization of private insurance to those who don't qualify for Medicaid are the largest changes that result from the law, reforms of the health insurance market ultimately could have the biggest impact on the health financing system. There are currently three distinct private markets for insurance in the USA. The large group market functions reasonably well. The vast majority of large employers offer their workers health insurance, and whether self or fully insured, there is a reasonably efficient market for purchasing these services.

In contrast, the small group and individual markets are broken. These are markets that are used by small employers or individuals, and they suffer from a problem common to many insurance markets called adverse selection. Because individuals without insurance previously have not been compelled to purchase coverage, those who seek to purchase coverage usually have a greater need for insurance than the average person. For instance, healthy 30-year-olds frequently forgo purchasing coverage until they either develop a serious condition or suffer an injury. Recognizing this possibility, insurance companies often prevent individuals from obtaining coverage when they have a medical condition or price the insurance assuming such an event will occur. A consequence of adverse selection is that insurance for individuals and some small businesses are expensive that it prevents even those who are healthier from obtaining coverage.

Health insurance companies have developed a variety of strategies to deal with adverse selection, including intensive medical underwriting, whereby policies are priced based on risks that are known at the time of purchase, limits or delays in coverage for preexisting conditions, and very high prices. The ACA makes several changes that will substantially improve these markets over time. Many young people oppose the ACA, believing it will just make it more expensive for them to buy insurance, whereas these changes are likely to result in improved affordability in these formerly dysfunctional markets for several reasons.

First, because of the individual mandate, insurers participating in these markets now have fewer concerns about adverse selection. Although some have questioned whether the penalties for not adhering to the mandate are too small to force compliance, in Massachusetts similar-sized penalties have proven sufficient [9, 10]. Second, these markets will no longer use individual medical underwriting, but rather will standardize pricing within age and sex bands so as to not price sicker individuals out of the market. Although young and healthy individuals will be paying somewhat more than is actuarially needed, as they grow older and inevitably sicker, the subsequent lower rates will more than compensate. Also many thousands of individuals at all ages will now be able to obtain more coverage at affordable rates.

Fixing this market also should provide a psychological safety net to most people who fear that losing their job will result in losing their health insurance coverage. This is a particular concern for those with chronic medical conditions such as diabetes or heart disease who would have been priced out of the individual market. Now, those who lose their employer-sponsored coverage will have options that did not exist before. Reform of this market will also go a long way towards eliminating what has been called "job lock." Currently, the individual and small group markets are seen as a significant impediment to entrepreneurs and others wanting to leave a large employer to start their own companies. Previously, concerns about not being able to obtain health insurance coverage might have caused them to stay at their current jobs. Thus, the fixing of this market also should improve job mobility for those with employer-sponsored insurance. In short, a functioning insurance market serves as an important underlying safety net.

Third, states also have the option to actively manage their insurance exchanges as active purchasers of care. Although not all states will choose to set up their exchanges in this manner, the experiences of the Massachusetts Connector suggest that the exchange can play an important role in facilitating comparisons across plans and in exacting lower premium increases [11]. To the extent that exchanges force plans to conform to relative standard levels of coverage, this will facilitate comparisons among plans and make the market more accessible for average consumers.

There also are a number of insurance coverage-related aspects of the ACA that generally are without controversy and support of these features is nearly universal. For instance, adult children can now remain on their parent's insurance policy until the age of 26. Although generally well, adults in this age range often lacked employer-sponsored insurance and frequently lacked insurance because they could not afford to purchase coverage in the individual market. Yet, extending insurance to this population is relatively inexpensive when concerns of adverse selection are mitigated. Thus, this simple change extended insurance coverage to approximately three million individuals at a relatively low cost to all [12].

Similarly, eliminating the "donut hole" or lack of coverage for seniors that have extensive prescription drug expenses but less than catastrophic expenses is currently part of Medicare's prescription drug coverage. The donut hole is widely seen as problematic, leading to nonadherence and difficulty affording medications for vulnerable elderly enrollees taking multiple medications. Closing the donut hole, which will be accomplished by 2019, is largely without controversy, as are the intermediate steps being taken in that direction over the next several years.

Elimination of lifetime caps on insurance plans ultimately will affect few people but will have a big positive impact on a few. Finally, assuring that all health insurance plans include minimum acceptable benefits (i.e., essential benefits) is also seen as attractive to most people and should make it easier for individuals to evaluate insurance products since many will offer relatively standard benefits without the exceptions hidden in small print that previously were common.

Delivery System Reorganization Is the Ultimate Prize

The continued rise in healthcare costs is seen as a threat to the viability of the US economy. Health costs are consuming ever-larger portions of government budgets, including local, state, and the federal government and crowding out other spending [13]. In the private sector, growth in the amount that employers pay for employer-sponsored health insurance has accounted for most of their increases in employee compensation since 2000, leaving most individuals and families with less discretionary income to spend on other goods.

There has been much criticism of the ACA and its failure to control healthcare cost growth explicitly. Although there is some validity to these criticisms in the short run, over time the ACA will be a powerful force to lower healthcare costs that are ultimately needed for the healthcare system to be sustainable. Moreover, it would be inaccurate to say that the ACA left the issue of cost control for the future. The act contains numerous provisions and experiments that will be useful in tackling cost control in the coming years. These include the establishment of the Patient Centered Outcomes Research Institute (PCORI) to better define the comparative effectiveness of various approaches to care and the funding of the Centers for Medicare and Medicaid Innovation with approximately $1 billion per year to encourage new forms of healthcare delivery systems. In addition, the act specified important programs related to global payments such as the accountable care organization (ACO) program as well as experimentation with various forms of primary care payment reform that ultimately will be useful under a redesigned healthcare delivery system.

Finally, by providing coverage for the uninsured, it will be easier and fairer to spread the burdens of less spending across the entire population. Controlling costs will require cutting funding from many components of the system. To do this fairly it is important that most individuals be covered and that the coverage playing field be relatively level.

It should come as no surprise that Massachusetts, which established almost universal coverage for all its citizens several years ago, is the first state in the country to deal with the challenges of controlling the total cost of care within the state. As part of its 2006 health reform, which served as a model for the ACA, the state subsidized the purchase of private insurance for those whose income was below a threshold and required those above the threshold to buy health insurance coverage from the private market. The legislation further established a statewide health insurance exchange called the Connector to facilitate the purchase of insurance for these groups. The prices faced by those purchasing insurance would now be easily known to all throughout the state. Since the state was subsidizing the purchase of insurance or mandating that citizens obtain this coverage themselves, it provided a strong incentive for the state to play an active role in seeing that future premiums were affordable and not growing at excessive rates. Thus, controlling rising costs became a central concern of the government in a way that it was not prior to the implementation of health reform.

This pressure in Massachusetts accomplished two notable results. First, the growth in costs of insurance offered over the exchange has been substantially lower than that seen in other states across the country [14]. In fact, in comparison to the rest of the United States, non-group premiums for family and single plans in Massachusetts experienced 52 % and 35 % slower growth, respectively. And second, Massachusetts just passed comprehensive cost control legislation that sets a benchmark for the future growth in all healthcare spending in the state [15]. This benchmark was set initially to correspond to the yearly growth in the state's income (analogous to the state GDP). To avoid short-term fluctuations in the economy, the benchmark reflects the yearly growth in the state's potential income. To accomplish this goal, the state is relying on several changes that have recently been made in the way healthcare is paid for and delivered in the private market. The state will carefully monitor the progress of these private initiatives and help support their implementation. For those payers and providers that resist improving, the state has authorized an independent commission to require such changes or levy fines. Not surprising, Massachusetts healthcare providers lead the country in the adoption of global payment and other delivery system reforms [16, 17].

Finally, although providing insurance and health care is expensive, preventive services aimed at maintaining the health of the population are among the services with the greatest value. With all now covered under the blanket of coverage, the ACA allows the system to reorganize itself around the provision of adequate primary and preventive care to maintain the health of the population, rather than focusing on expensive acute treatments for conditions that may have been prevented with adequate prevention. Moreover, these important preventive services are now covered in full under the ACA.

Conclusions

The ACA is a monumental piece of legislation that represents the single most important set of reforms to the health system since the establishment of Medicare and Medicaid in 1965. Although many object to some of its provisions, the Act achieves major accomplishments by extending health coverage to millions of Americans, enacting much needed reforms of private insurance market and putting in place numerous provisions that over time represent the best options of controlling the inexorable growth in the costs of providing healthcare to US citizens. Moreover, the status quo that many long for is likely an illusion, as accelerating rates of loss of private insurance coverage that had been present prior to enactment would likely have continued unabated. While there is much that is unknown about the impact of the ACA, lessons from Massachusetts and other experiments in payment and delivery reform suggest that most Americans stand to benefit from its passage.

Nonetheless, significant challenges related to insurance coverage remain, particularly given the large number of states that have elected to forgo expansion of their Medicaid programs.

References

1. Buettgens M, Hall M. Who will be uninsured after health insurance reform? Robert Wood Johnson Foundation; 2011.
2. Status of State Action on the Medicaid Expansion Decision, as of July 1, 2013. Kaiser Family Foundation.http://www.kff.org/medicaid/state-indicator/state-activity-around-expanding-medicaid-under-the-affordable-care-act/. Accessed on July 12, 2013.
3. Kaiser Family Foundation. Health Tracking Poll: November 2012; 2012.
4. Kaiser Family Foundation. Health tracking poll: march 2011; 2011.
5. Schoen C, Doty MM, Robertson RH, Collins SR. Affordable Care Act reforms could reduce the number of underinsured US adults by 70 percent. Health Aff. 2011;30:1762–71.
6. Organization for Economic Co-Operation and Development (OECD). OECD health data 2012; 2012.
7. Kenney GM, Dubay L, Zuckerman S, Huntress M. Opting out of the Medicaid expansion under the ACA: How many uninsured adults would not be eligible for Medicaid? Washington, DC: Urban Institute; 2012.
8. http://kaiserfamilyfoundation.files.wordpress.com/2013/07/8458-analyzing-the-impact-of-state-medicaid-expansion-decisions2.pdf.
9. Wilensky GR. The shortfalls of Obamacare. N Engl J Med. 2012;367(16):1479–81.
10. Doonan MT, Tull KR. Health care reform in Massachusetts: implementation of coverage expansions and a health insurance mandate. Milbank Q. 2010;88:54–80.
11. Kingsdale J. Health insurance exchanges—key link in a better-value chain. N Engl J Med. 2010;362:2147–50.
12. Sommers BD, Schwartz K. 2.5 million young adults gain health insurance due to the Affordable Care Act. Office of the Assistant Secretary for Planning and Evaluation, Department of Health and Human Services; 2011:1.
13. Chernew ME, Baicker K, Hsu J. The specter of financial armageddon- health care and federal debt in the United States. N Engl J Med. 2010;362:1166–8.
14. Graves JA, Gruber J. How did health care reform in Massachusetts impact insurance premiums? Am Econ Rev. 2012;102:508–13.
15. Chapter 224 of the Acts of 2012, An act improving the quality of health care and reducing costs through increased transparency, efficiency and innovation; 2012 (Accessed 2012).
16. Song Z, Landon BE. Controlling health care spending—the Massachusetts experiment. N Engl J Med. 2012;366:1560–1.
17. Ayanian JZ, Van der Wees PJ. Tackling rising health care costs in Massachusetts. N Engl J Med. 2012;367:790–3.

Chapter 12
Messaging, Medicine, and Obamacare

Ceci Connolly

A messaging guru might well caution that calling the Affordable Care Act (ACA) an "experiment" conjures up images of lab rats and guinea pigs, and that the American people might not like the idea that something with so much potential to affect their daily lives is an experiment with an uncertain outcome. To scientists and clinicians, "experiment" is a word laden with positive value. To most of the general public, the idea of human health experiments is terrifying.

As a journalist covering the drafting and passage of the ACA, I saw the Obama administration and Democratic senators wrestling daily with how to talk about healthcare reform. An age-old maxim says that it is easier to tear down than to build, so perhaps the Republicans were always going to have an easier time vilifying the ACA than the Democrats were going to have promoting it. But it may be instructive to trace the course of the controversy about healthcare reform in 2009–2010 and, since then, to see what did and did not resonate with the public and what this may suggest about the public's ultimate attitude toward the ACA.

If we look at public attitudes toward healthcare reform from October 2008 through August 2009, we can see that positive reception began to wane in conjunction with a decline in the president's favorability ratings. The percentages of Americans who said that it was more important than ever to reform healthcare and those who said we couldn't afford to do so closely tracked President Barack Obama's favorability ratings over the same period (Fig. 12.1).

The numbers show that President Obama and his signature healthcare initiative enjoyed the honeymoon with the public that every newly elected president gets. No one was more cognizant of this phenomenon than Rahm Emanuel, who was then White House chief of staff and who would undoubtedly have liked the healthcare bill to move to a vote about March 1, 2009, if that had been possible. For every

C. Connolly, BA (✉)
Former National Health Correspondent, Washington Post, DC, USA
e-mail: connollyceci@gmail.com

H.P. Selker and J.S. Wasser (eds.), *The Affordable Care Act as a National Experiment:*   99
Health Policy Innovations and Lessons, DOI 10.1007/978-1-4614-8351-9_12,
© Springer Science+Business Media New York 2014

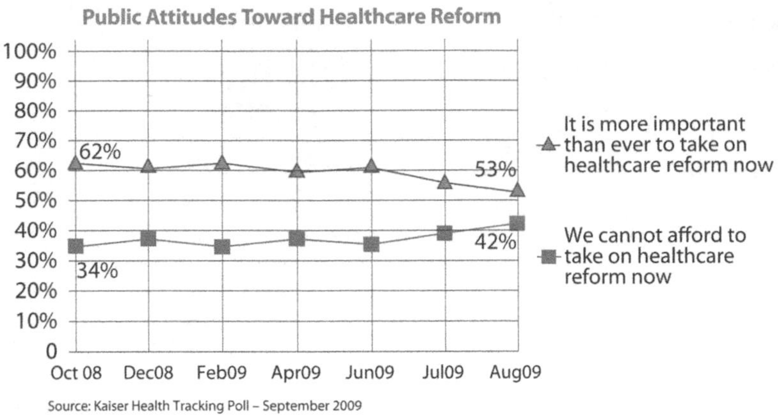

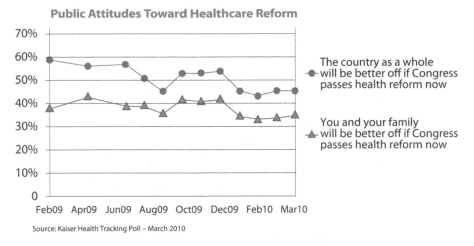

Fig. 12.1 Public support for health reform declines during the heat of the debate. (Reproduced with permission from the Kaiser Health Tracking Poll, September 2009. Kaiser Family Foundation, 2009)

Fig. 12.2 As public support for health reform waivers, many believe there is a greater public benefit than personal benefit. (Reproduced with permission from the Kaiser Health Tracking Poll, March 2010. Kaiser Family Foundation, 2010)

administration, things get a lot more challenging when it comes time to govern rather than simply campaign.

Not surprisingly then, support for healthcare reform fell from its high of 62 % right after Barack Obama's inauguration as president to 56 % in July 2009. And then it fell even further to 53 % in August 2009. A lot has been written about public attitudes toward healthcare reform in March 2010 when the bill was passed in Congress and signed by the president. But my hypothesis is that the message war was actually lost from Memorial Day to Labor Day 2009.

A Kaiser Family Foundation poll offers another snapshot of public attitudes during the time between President Obama's inauguration and the passage of the ACA (Figs. 12.2 and 12.3).

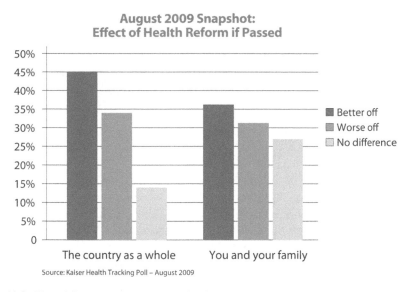

Fig. 12.3 The public perceives greater benefit of health reform to the country as a whole and less for them and their families. (Reproduced with permission from the Kaiser Health Tracking Poll, August 2009. Kaiser Family Foundation, 2009)

The different responses to two questions posed in August 2009—whether the country as a whole would be better or worse off and whether you and your family would be better or worse off if the healthcare reform passed—reflect a common, perhaps universal, human phenomenon. It goes something like this. Ask people if they like their congressman and they say, "Oh, yes. Yes, indeed. He's such a nice guy. He's wonderful." Ask people what they think of the Congress and they say, "I can't stand those dirty bastards. They're terrible. Throw them all out of office."

A similar thing occurs when it comes to healthcare. Ask people what they think of their own doctor and they say, "My doctor is wonderful. He always listens to me. He's so kind." Ask people what they think of the healthcare system and they say, "It's a mess. It's too expensive. I can't stand the insurers. Doctors are arrogant and cold. Hospital food is terrible," and so on.

It is just human nature that we want and need to believe that those we personally rely on as representatives, and even more so those we personally rely on as healers, are special. It is the way humans think and feel. It is how we react to and judge circumstances.

Thus when the Kaiser Family Foundation asked people in August 2009 if the country as a whole would be better off if healthcare reform passed, 45 % said yes. But when the foundation asked people if you and your family would be better off if healthcare reform passed, only 36 % said yes. There are divergent views when people focus on their own circumstances versus everyone else's.

The divergence in the Kaiser Family Foundation data is so telling, because the majority of Americans get health insurance through their employers. The so-called Hillary Care failed in President Bill Clinton's first term because people were

Why is Max Baucus Even a Democrat?

By Paul Horgarth, Sept 16, 2009

Fig. 12.4 Contentious headlines mar the healthcare debate and illustrate the lack of bipartisanship. (Reproduced with permission from Hogarth, P. Beyond Chron, September 16, 2009)

concerned that they were going to lose what they had. The "Harry and Louise" commercials from the Health Insurance Association of America made people associate "Hillary Care" with losing their health insurance, and we see a similar concern in the Kaiser Family Foundation's August 2009 polling.

Another important point to remember is that Barack Obama did not campaign in 2008 on a healthcare-for-all platform. That was John Edwards; that was Hillary Clinton. They supported an individual mandate. Barack Obama opposed an individual mandate. The only thing candidate Obama initially wanted to say about healthcare was that he would lower Americans' healthcare costs. And so when Obama became president, most Americans thought that his healthcare promise was that costs were going to go down.

Of course, it's impossible to lower healthcare costs. You might be able to slow the rate of growth, but there's no way you're ever going to lower healthcare costs by a penny.

With the polling data on public attitudes to healthcare in mind, let's look at a headline from the long hot summer of 2009, from the San Francisco-based, progressive news website BeyondChron.org (Fig. 12.4).

As action on the healthcare reform bill slowed in the summer of 2009, Max Baucus, then chairman of the Senate Finance Committee, was trying very hard to build bipartisan support for the bill in that committee. Although progressives excoriated him for this, bipartisan support was an admirable goal and one that used to be achievable on Capitol Hill. Democrats and Republicans used to compromise fairly often on tax and budget policy, trade policy, and most of all foreign policy, especially in the Senate. And so Max Baucus spent the long hot summer in truly interminable meetings with staffers, Republican members of the finance committee, and his fellow Democrats trying to fashion a compromise on healthcare reform.

Unfortunately, outside of Congress there were Democratic congressmen, such as Maryland's Frank Kratovil, hanging in effigy because of their association with healthcare reform. That indicated a level of partisan political rancor that made compromise inside Congress impossible (Fig. 12.5).

The Republican on the Senate Finance Committee that Max Baucus was trying hardest to woo was Chuck Grassley of Iowa. Chuck Grassley got countless meetings with Max Baucus. Chuck Grassley got invited to the White House to have a hamburger lunch with the president. In response to all this solicitous attention from the Democrats, Grassley told an August town hall meeting in Iowa, "We should not have a government program that determines if you're going to pull the plug on grandma." That prospect, the notion that healthcare reform would create so-called death panels, was the real downfall of the Democrats in the message war.

Fig. 12.5 An example
of partisan infighting over
healthcare reform. Courtesy
of Joe Albero, http://www.
sbynews.com

Rep. Frank Kratovil (D-MD) in Effigy

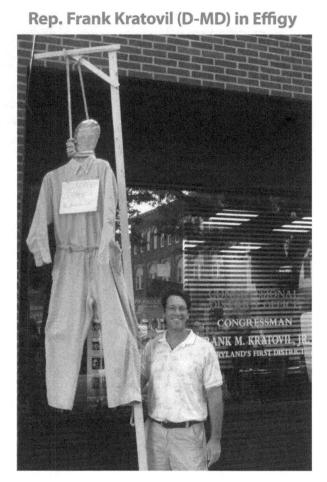

There were never going to be death panels. But the Obama White House was slow to say it that simply and that forcefully. The foundering of Michael Dukakis's 1988 presidential campaign as it failed to rebut criticism from the Republicans had taught Democrats not to let attacks go unanswered, and during the Clinton years they showed they'd learned this lesson. But in 2009 they seemed to have temporarily forgotten it.

When the Republicans started talking about death panels, all of my sources in the White House said, "This is so ridiculous, nobody could possibly believe it. We do not have to even respond, because it is so absurd. We don't want to elevate this notion." For a day or two I thought they might be right, because that's the way the mainstream media used to behave as well. Newspaper editors did not give outrageous falsehoods additional credibility by headlining them on the front page. Television news programs did not lead their reports with them. But that quaint period is long past.

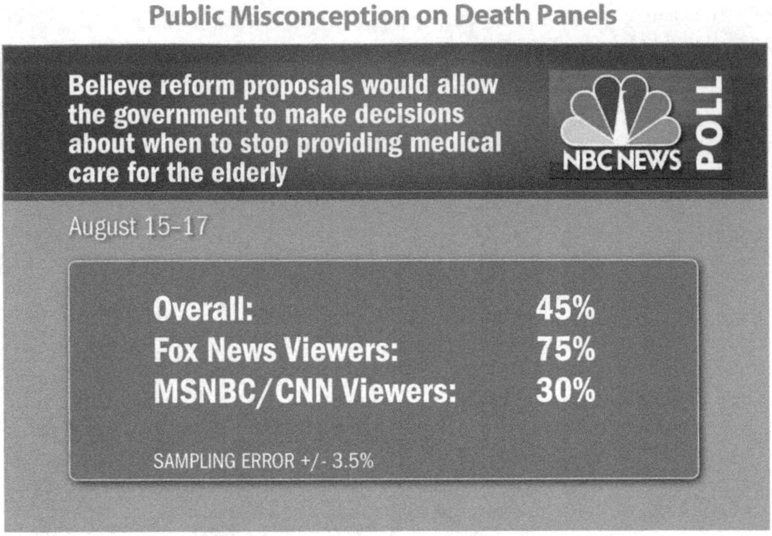

Public Misconception on Death Panels

Believe reform proposals would allow
the government to make decisions
about when to stop providing medical
care for the elderly

NBC NEWS POLL

August 15–17

Overall: 45%
Fox News Viewers: 75%
MSNBC/CNN Viewers: 30%

SAMPLING ERROR +/- 3.5%

Fig. 12.6 Conservatives in particular buy into the concept of "death panels" propagated by opponents of the law. (Courtesy of NBCUniversal Archives)

The result was that in August 2009 a great many Americans believed that healthcare reform was going to create death panels. This was especially so if they were Fox News viewers (Fig. 12.6).

A full 75 % of Fox News viewers believed that healthcare reform meant the government was going to have death panels. But we shouldn't miss the fact that 30 % of MSNBC and CNN viewers, and 45 % of Americans overall, believed the same thing.

The lesson here is that healthcare is very complicated and very personal. There was after all a kernel of truth to the alleged prospect of death panels. The legislation as then written was in fact going to permit Medicare to pay for a counseling session with a physician to discuss end-of-life choices. In trying to explain and justify this, the proponents of healthcare reform tumbled, like Alice in Wonderland, down into the rhetorical looking glass.

The more those in favor of reform talked about end-of-life counseling and how helpful it would be, the more they triggered discomfort in people's minds about the very difficult decisions they might have to make about their own lives or the lives of family members—and the more and more confused average Americans became about just what healthcare reform was going to do. When issues get personal, and there obviously is no issue more personal than health and healthcare, the discussion suddenly becomes very, very complicated.

Again, end-of-life counseling was never going to be the death panel scenario that opponents of healthcare reform portrayed. If end-of-life counseling were commonplace, it would surely help limit a lot of unnecessary suffering, physical and mental, that people and their families go through as the end of life approaches.

An illustration of the fact that life-and-death issues are never simple or clean emerged when President Obama tried to use his maternal grandmother's experience as a teaching moment for the nation on healthcare reform. In an April 2009 interview with the *New York Times*, the president revealed that shortly before the election the previous November, his 86-year-old grandmother, Madelyn Dunham, chose to have a hip replacement despite a prior diagnosis that she had terminal cancer. Her condition worsened after the hip replacement surgery, and she died two days before the election.

President Obama told the *New York Times*, "I would have paid out of pocket for that hip replacement, just because she's my grandmother. Whether, sort of in the aggregate, society making those decisions to give my grandmother, or everybody else's aging grandparents or parents, a hip replacement when they're terminally ill is a sustainable model, is a very difficult question" [1].

The labored phrasing and syntax of that last sentence, coming from someone as justly renowned for being articulate as Barack Obama is, indicate how difficult the messaging on healthcare reform was for the Democrats in 2009. Navigating the gap between the personal and "sort of in the aggregate" is hard emotionally, intellectually, and rhetorically.

As someone who wants to be a responsible healthcare consumer, I wondered if my 72-year-old mother should have both knees replaced on Medicare's dime. My mother now plays golf three days a week, and she outdrives me on the course. She has a full life. So again, healthcare is complicated because it is personal and it is individualized. Every time you think you've come up with some good guide posts for how to move forward, along comes someone like my mother who can drive a ball 200 yards and has great quality of life because of her knee replacements, and she has just tossed your guidepost out the window.

That's why the messaging gets so very challenging. That's why it was so ironic that in August 2009 political pundits and cartoonists were riffing on the Republicans' attack line, "Obama wants to pull the plug on grandma!" He hadn't pulled the plug on medical care for his own grandmother, but he was attacked as if he hypocritically wanted to pull the plug on medical care for the nation's grandmothers. And none of his characteristically nuanced attempts to balance opposing concerns on the issue—in that same interview with the *New York Times* he said, "If somebody told me that my grandmother couldn't have a hip replacement and she had to lie there in misery in her waning days—that would be pretty upsetting"—got through to the public.

If we want to explain how the Democrats lost the messaging war on healthcare reform in 2009, aside from the fact that messaging is a difficult challenge to begin with, I think there are two other theories to consider.

The first is that the Democrats missed their opportunity in the summer of 2009. They had 60 votes in the Senate, a filibuster-proof majority. They still had a relatively popular president. The recession hadn't dragged on so long that everyone was pessimistic about the future. So the Democrats could have moved the bill. They simply could have moved it through, LBJ style. They had the votes. It would have been done. You wouldn't have had healthcare reform hanging in the balance until after the death of Ted Kennedy, with Republican Scott Brown being elected to fill the empty Senate seat from Massachusetts. That meant the reform bill had to be completed through a process known as budget reconciliation, which only required 51 votes in the Senate. The maneuver enabled Democrats to enact the bill, but they could not use a traditional "conference committee" to address holes in the early version of the bill. The second theory is that in some respects the messaging wasn't all bad. One decision that I believe was very effective and important for the passage of the ACA was that the Obama administration took great pains to demonize the healthcare industry. The administration was criticized by progressives for that, but Obama and his advisors came to healthcare with the mistakes of "Hillary Care" fresh in their minds. And from a practical point of view, they were wise to remember that the insurance industry's "Harry and Louise" television commercials helped scuttle reform in the 1990s.

There is evidence to suggest that Americans do know what's in the ACA. And what they know is that in the near term it is mostly about access to healthcare for those who are now uninsured. Yes, there are some good quality measures in the law. There are some promising but small initiatives in the direction of controlling costs, which over time hold out the promise of making inroads on both cost and quality. But in reality, in the early years of this legislation, it is about access.

The ACA as written, passed, and signed was going to address access in two ways: through an expansion of Medicaid and through subsidies for purchasing health insurance on state exchanges or a fallback federal exchange. In late June 2012, the Supreme Court ruled that the Medicaid expansion is optional for states, but it left the remainder of the law intact including the new health insurance exchanges. Thus the ACA will still expand coverage in a very substantial way.

Up to 27 million Americans are projected to receive coverage through this legislation. The American electorate historically has been slow to embrace universal-access initiatives, especially any that involve taxpayer dollars and in a persistently weak economy. It is hardly surprising that people's attitudes and votes reflect their own self-interest. So as voters, especially those who already have health insurance, came to understand that the ACA is first and foremost about access for the uninsured, their support for the legislation fell. In a March 2010 Kaiser Family Foundation poll on the effect of passage of the ACA, 45 % said the country as a whole would be better off while only 35 % said their family would be better off (Figs. 12.2 and 12.3). During that same time, a Gallup poll conducted in mid-March 2010 showed that people understood the benefits of the bill—59 % said it would make things better for Americans who did not have health insurance—but did not necessarily see the benefits of the bill for the country as a whole or for their own families. Thirty-nine percent said it would make things better for the nation as a whole, and only 28 % said it would make things better for them and their families. It was less a case of bad messaging than unpopularity for legislation aimed at a distinct minority.

If we are guided by history, we need not obsess over the polling. Americans are fickle. They change their minds often. Politically, for some time now, the country has been changing its mind every two years in terms of which party gets control of the Congress.

In addition, as much as people don't like change and are resistant to change, they are also incredibly resilient. A look at our healthcare policy history shows that major changes such as the creation of Medicare in 1965 and the more recent addition of the Medicare Part D prescription drug program were unpopular when they were first passed. Today there is no doubt that Medicare overall and the Part D prescription drug program are exceedingly popular. Yes, they have gone through tweaks, changes, improvements, and expansions. They regularly need to be modernized and changed. But in terms of public opinion, it largely comes down to this: we are all human and change is scary. But we are also resilient.

We know that the healthcare landscape is changing—quickly and dramatically. The Affordable Care Act injects some energy and money into the transformation of the system, but fundamentally it is not the cause of sweeping change. Economic realities such as the unsustainable growth trajectory of health spending and increased demands for true value are the root drivers of the change. And regardless of the ACA, those forces are not going away any time soon.

Reference

1. Leonhardt, D. After the Great Recession. New York Times, 2009; April 28.

Part IV
From Personal to Political to Policy: What Next?

Chapter 13
Commentary on Part IV: From Personal to Political to Policy—What Next?

James Roosevelt, Jr., Terence Burke, and Paul Jean

We hear the term "Obamacare" used more often now to refer to the Affordable Care Act (ACA). It's spoken with derision by critics while supporters used to recoil when they heard it. I embrace the term and say it freely because, as a supporter of the Affordable Care Act, I believe that this is a remarkable public policy accomplishment that will forever define President Obama's tenure, just as Social Security did FDR's and Medicare Lyndon Johnson's.

While it marks a major milestone in America's public policy history, we must remember that the ACA is not the final goal of universal healthcare but rather a significant foundation for programs and policies that will continue to move this nation forward to universal healthcare coverage.

Since the late 1800s, America has been wrestling with putting in place some system to provide people with affordable healthcare coverage. Until the passage of the ACA, each attempt was either scuttled early on due to political pressure or failed in its legislative infancy. Fortunately, this country did manage to pass important programs like Medicare and Medicaid to cover our most vulnerable populations. But, we remained far behind most of the industrial world in terms of providing healthcare coverage to all of our population.

The ACA creates a framework for significant reform of the way healthcare is organized, delivered, and paid for. It will also result in sweeping changes to the business practices of health insurers and a significant expansion of private and public health insurance coverage.

J. Roosevelt, Jr., JD (✉)
Tufts Health Plan, Watertown, MA, USA
e-mail: James_roosevelt@tufts-health.com

T. Burke • P. Jean
Denterlein, Boston, MA, USA
e-mail: tburke@denterlein.com; pjean@denterlein.com

H.P. Selker and J.S. Wasser (eds.), *The Affordable Care Act as a National Experiment:*
Health Policy Innovations and Lessons, DOI 10.1007/978-1-4614-8351-9_13,
© Springer Science+Business Media New York 2014

Having survived the gauntlet of legal and legislative challenges that have come its way, the ACA will have a greater impact on more people than perhaps any law in American history.

Aside from the effects on changing the healthcare industry, the passage of the ACA also enshrines a more significant role for government in providing access to healthcare—like it or not. With the president's initiative, Congress's action, and the Supreme Court's ruling, all three branches of government agreed that *something* must and could be done to address the issues of access, quality, and cost—and that represents a huge achievement for this country.

As Shawn Bishop points out in her piece, "Supreme Court Review of the Affordable Care Act and Political Gamesmanship," before the oral arguments, those in government and the healthcare community believed the ACA would survive the review by the Supreme Court because a "large body of settled law and previous Supreme Court rulings seemed to indicate that the court, no matter how divided it might be, would have little choice but to uphold the ACA." This highlights the fact that the ACA is built on a very strong foundation created over years of incremental movement toward government playing a larger role in the guarantee of healthcare coverage. It wasn't until the oral arguments, which featured a sharp tone and tough questioning by the justices, that serious doubts began to be raised by both sides that the law would pass constitutional muster.

However, that was not to be.

The majority decision delivered by Chief Justice John Roberts caught almost all observers by surprise especially because none of the permutations of possible outcomes that Shawn Bishop says prognosticators put forward came true. In fact, the Court delivered what was perhaps the least probable outcome when it issued two key decisions upholding the individual mandate while striking down the law's provision making *all* federal funding of a state's Medicaid program conditional on the state's agreeing to implement the significant expansion of Medicaid coverage.

The Court ruled that Congress could not require individuals to purchase health insurance on the basis of its authority under the Commerce Clause. However, it upheld the mandate as an exercise of Congress's taxing power, asserting that since the only consequence of an individual not maintaining health insurance is making an additional payment to the IRS, the mandate was, in fact, a tax.

A close reading of history tells us that we should not have been too surprised by the Court's decision to protect the individual mandate as a tax. Even past Supreme Court majorities, which were inclined to reign in federal power, have given broader latitude to Congress under its taxing authority than under the Commerce Clause. The Court, for example, first initially upheld major New Deal enactments on the basis of Congress's power to tax.

Shawn Bishop makes an interesting observation in her piece that if Congress and the president had originally called the penalty a tax, the case that came before the Supreme Court would have never made its way through the lower courts. However, if it had been referred to as a tax in the development of the legislation, it would never have passed Congress. We are fortunate that the Court saw the mandate properly and upheld the law and protected the mandate, which is vital to the ACA's effectiveness.

As for its ruling on the Medicaid expansion, the Court's decision was a radical departure from its own precedent. The ACA enlarges the population covered by Medicaid to include adults under age 65 earning up to 133 % of the poverty level. However, the Court, by a 7-2 margin, found that the provision by which Congress threatened to withhold existing Medicaid funds from states which refused to accept the Medicaid expansion was "impermissibly coercive."

While this ruling agreed with the briefs filed by Attorneys General from 26 states, it struck many legal scholars as unusual given that the Court has long upheld Congress' power to regulate how it spends the money it provides to programs—in this case Medicaid. Justice Ginsburg pointed out in her dissent that this was "the first time ever [that the Court] finds an exercise of Congress's spending power unconstitutionally coercive." However, I and others believe that when reluctant states see the value in expanding Medicaid and the transfer of tax dollars to participating states, this part of the ruling will prove to be much less damaging to the ACA's goals than it appears today.

When the Supreme Court effectively made the Medicaid expansion optional for states, several Republican-controlled states expressed strong opposition to moving forward with the expansion even though it would bring relief to many of their residents who are in need. No doubt, this stance had much to do with political posturing before the 2012 elections. As of this writing, 24 states are moving forward with Medicaid expansion, 21 are not moving forward, and six are debating it, according to the Kaiser Family Foundation. The question now is whether the hold-out governors or legislatures will continue to oppose Medicaid expansion or whether they will succumb to logic and public pressure to accept additional federal funding.

Although these governors and legislators claim that the Medicaid expansion places a significant burden on the states, the truth is, it does not. The federal government will pay 100 % of the costs for newly eligible adults between 2014 and 2016. States will start to contribute beginning in 2017, but their share would top out at 10 % in 2020 and thereafter. In fact, states will gain largely from replacing state and local spending on uncompensated care and mental health services.

In the "limbo" period leading up to the presidential election, some states said they were holding out against establishing the health insurance exchanges mandated by the ACA. However, in many of those states, officials were quietly beginning to put together the framework for the exchanges in order to meet deadlines for informing the federal government if the state would establish and operate its own exchange. The strong desire to keep out the federal government is proving to be a strong incentive for states that oppose the exchanges. As Donald Hughes, the healthcare policy adviser to Governor Jan Brewer of Arizona, told the New York Times," If we have to have one, then it would be better for Arizona to do it ourselves rather than defer to the federal government." Today, 17 states have their own exchanges, seven are planning for Partnership Exchanges, the state-federal hybrid, and 27 are defaulting to the federal government establishing their exchange. With the ACA firmly ensconced as federal law, the creation and conversations around the exchanges will further solidify the role of government in providing access to healthcare in the public's mind.

As we have seen with the major health insurance reforms which became effective soon after the ACA's passage, the law will become even more rooted and stable as the most far-reaching elements of the law become effective at the beginning of 2014. As the ACA works to expand access to care and bring change to people's lives and as its pilot programs and public-private partnerships begin to reshape the healthcare market and stabilize rising healthcare costs, those results will further solidify the ACA's standing and codify the government's role in the delivery of healthcare with the public and politicians.

This will take time however. And, in fact, the ACA is really only a part of a much larger set of changes occurring at the federal, state, and market levels that are shaping the future of what we call "healthcare reform."

John McDonough frames this viewpoint coherently in his chapter, "Next Experiments in ACA Legislation and Policy." As McDonough states, "If we look at the ACA as part of the broad goal of making American healthcare equal to that in the rest of the developed world in fairness, patient outcomes, and population health, those of us who favor reform must recognize that the struggle for reform will play out over the next decade, if not longer."

The ACA is already acting as a powerful accelerant that is beginning to reorient the healthcare system toward a greater emphasis on prevention and keeping the population healthy, reform the healthcare delivery system, and focus on wellness and health outcomes. In the end, these provisions may be as significant as the expansion of access to healthcare in terms of improving the health of the American people.

While government is a major driver of these steps in healthcare reform, at least at the federal level and in a couple of states including Massachusetts, the market, especially the health insurance sector, is making significant progress in advancing health reform and improving the health of people. For instance, in Massachusetts, health insurers have been moving providers toward more risk-based payment systems, known as global payments, and away from fee-for-service that perpetuates higher costs. This not only controls rising costs by targeting care more efficiently, it also improves the coordination of care by encouraging better management by the primary care physician and more communication among the doctors in a patient's care group, which leads to better health outcomes. Improvement in the quality of care is addressed as well in the move to global payments as physicians are held to quality standards and outcomes as part of their contract with payers.

Private companies have stepped up their commitment to providing wellness programs for their employees. Insurers are making a greater commitment than ever to study and improve wellness programs and make them available to employers and members.

If the market and government continue working as hard as they've been toward achieving the stages of healthcare reform laid out by John McDonnough, we will begin to see even more benefits in the form of cost stabilization and better health outcomes—the very reason why we've been striving for healthcare reform for so long.

John McDonough and I share the same perspective on the Massachusetts model of healthcare having both been actively involved in the creation of the state's landmark 2006 healthcare reform law. As the model for the ACA, the experience in Massachusetts bodes well for federal reform.

The Massachusetts experience further reinforces the importance of healthcare advocates remaining actively engaged in implementation of the healthcare law. Passage of the ACA is not the end point of healthcare reform. As John McDonough points out in his piece, "One thing Massachusetts shows is that the passage of near-universal coverage in 2006 did not lead people to go in a rabbit hole and say the problems of the system didn't matter anymore. If anything, it created a more urgent, realistic, and pragmatic conversation about cost containment." That conversation led to the passage of further cost containment laws in 2008, 2010, and 2012 that when combined with the changes going on in the market undertaken by payers and providers, have begun to significantly stabilize healthcare costs in Massachusetts.

The Massachusetts experience should also serve to dampen the hysteria being ginned by opponents of the ACA that the law will generate much higher taxes and is not fiscally sustainable. The Massachusetts Taxpayers Foundation, a moderately conservative business association, concluded in April 2012 that "Massachusetts has achieved near universal health coverage with only modest additional costs to state taxpayers."

Massachusetts residents today take it for granted that government plays an important role in providing access to healthcare. Whether people are poor, disabled, elderly, self-employed, or an employee of a small business, or that small business owner, they know that government will have a solution for healthcare access if they are in need. We can look forward to a day when all citizens can feel the same way.

The journey this country has taken in searching for a solution to providing its citizens with healthcare passed a major milestone with the Affordable Care Act. And milestone is the correct term because the ACA is only one point on a long road we've traveled, and we still have many more miles to go to reach the goal of a comprehensive healthcare system in which our citizens are healthy and costs are in control.

The most important victory however in the passage of the ACA, and its subsequent political survival, is that increasingly the people of the United States are acknowledging the important role of government in ensuring they have access to high-quality affordable healthcare throughout their lifetime in the same way they believe in the promises created in Social Security and Medicare.

Chapter 14
Supreme Court Review of the ACA and Political Gamesmanship

Shawn Bishop

On the eve of the June 28, 2012, announcement of the Supreme Court's decision on the Affordable Care Act (ACA), official Washington DC was in a state of nervous calm. Two years, three months, and five days after the Act was signed into law, the decision that would determine the fate of key provisions intended to expand health insurance coverage to tens of millions of Americans was finally at hand. The Congress and the White House knew the decision could weaken the expansion of insurance coverage envisioned in the law and have a long-lasting effect on the public's view of healthcare reform in the USA. Healthcare industry stakeholders, their lawyers, and their consultants had been discussing for months all the possible permutations of the court's ruling in *National Federation of Independent Business v. Sebelius*.[1]

Before the oral arguments on March 26–28, 2012, a tenuous consensus had formed inside the Beltway that the Supreme Court would narrowly uphold the provisions of the law that were under review. Many constitutional lawyers, including a few conservative ones, had argued publicly that the Constitution was broad enough to sanction the insurance-related provisions that Congress wrote into the law. More confidence in a favorable court ruling prevailed with respect to a provision of the ACA that set the terms of federal support for an expansion of coverage under Medicaid.

After the oral arguments, which were widely felt by the law's supporters and critics alike to be a negative event for the ACA, those sentiments changed. As spring wore into summer, the view increasingly took hold that the Supreme Court would

---

[1] The National Federation of Independent Business, a lobbying group, and 26 states were the plaintiffs in the case, and Secretary of Health and Human Services Kathleen Sebelius, as the holder of the cabinet post whose responsibilities lay at the heart of the new law, was the nominal defendant.

S. Bishop, MPP (✉)
Marwood Group, Washington, DC, USA
e-mail: sbishop@marwoodgroup.com

H.P. Selker and J.S. Wasser (eds.), *The Affordable Care Act as a National Experiment:* 117
Health Policy Innovations and Lessons, DOI 10.1007/978-1-4614-8351-9_14,
© Springer Science+Business Media New York 2014

strike down the ACA provisions under legal challenge or perhaps even strike down the entire law. The court's decision revolved around four constitutional issues. The most important issue concerned the ACA's individual mandate, with a financial penalty for individuals who failed to buy health insurance. This penalty would be regulated and assessed by the Internal Revenue Service like a tax, but it was not referred to as a tax in the text of law. The key question at hand was whether the mandate exceeded Congress's authority, under the Constitution's Commerce Clause, "To regulate Commerce … among the several States," and its authority, under the Necessary and Proper Clause, "To make all laws which shall be necessary and proper for carrying into Execution the … Powers vested … in the Government of the United States."

If Congress had written the individual penalty as a tax, the law clearly would have fallen under its taxing powers, and this aspect of *National Federation of Independent Business v. Sebelius* would never have made its way through the lower court system to the Supreme Court. But because of President Obama's promise of no new taxes on the middle class during the 2008 presidential campaign, the Democratic-controlled Senate attached a "penalty" to the mandate rather than a "tax."

In addition, the 26 state attorneys general who filed briefs against the ACA did so on the grounds that the terms of the ACA provision to expand health insurance coverage under Medicaid was impermissibly coercive. States that chose not to accept the expansion faced a total loss of federal Medicaid funds at the discretion of the Secretary of Health and Human Services. Prior to oral arguments, most constitutional lawyers did not anticipate that this challenge would get very far, as the Supreme Court had long recognized Congress's authority to determine how federal funds were to be distributed to states.

The attorneys general used very powerful and colorful language in petitioning the Supreme Court to rule against the terms of the Medicaid expansion. One claim was that the possible loss of all Medicaid funds made the federal government like "a pickpocket who takes a wallet and gives the true owner the 'option' of agreeing to certain conditions to get it back or having it given to a stranger."

The two other issues the Supreme Court considered—the application of the legal doctrine known as severability and the relevance of the Anti-Injunction Act—had appeared to be less murky before the oral arguments.

The doctrine of severability would only come into play if the court struck down the individual mandate that was part of the fulcrum of the ACA reforms of the health insurance market. In that eventuality the question would be whether the individual mandate could be severed from the rest of the law. If severability were upheld, all the other provisions of the ACA would be allowed to stand even if the mandate were struck down.

If the Supreme Court ruled that the mandate penalty was effectively a tax, then the Anti-Injunction Act might come into play. This law states that no appeal can be made against a tax until it is actually collected. The Supreme Court thus had the option of decreeing that the mandate penalty was a tax and telling the opponents of the individual mandate to bring suit again in 2015, when the tax would first be levied.

Possible SCOTUS Rulings on ACA

Multiple permutations of a Court ruling were possible

Oral arguments were heard on March 26–28, 2012

Key Constitutional Issues		Possible Court Rulings
Individual Mandate	Whether individual mandate exceeds Congress' Commerce and Necessary and Proper Clause Authority	
Anti-Injunction Act	Whether provisions if any should be severed from ACA should the Court strike down the individual mandate	Uphold Mandate + Medicaid
Medicaid Expansion	Whether financial inducement to adopt Medicaid expansion is impermissibly coercive	Strike Mandate Only
		Strike Mandate + Related
Individual Mandate Severability	Whether Anti-Injunction Act prevents Court from addressing constitutional issues; Act says consumers cannot challenge a tax law until they have to pay it, which would not occur until 2015	Strike Mandate + Rest of Law

Fig. 14.1 Possible projected outcomes of SCOTUS rulings vary from upholding/striking key provisions of the law to upholding/striking the entire law. Source: based on analysis from the Marwood Group Advisory, LLC, 2012

There were many conceivable permutations to the court's ruling on these four questions. However, policymakers and healthcare stakeholders were most Focused on four scenarios (Fig. 14.1).

Of these four scenarios, one was that the Supreme Court would uphold the entire law, including the mandate and Medicaid expansion. A second possibility was that the court would strike down the mandate only. A third possibility was that the court would strike down the mandate plus certain related health insurance reform provisions, such as guaranteed issue (a prohibition on denying people coverage on the basis of preexisting conditions) and community rating (a prohibition on imposing differential rates based on individual health status). A fourth possibility was that the court would strike down the mandate and the rest of the law.

In addition to a palpable sentiment in Washington, DC, there was a thriving speculative market in these four possibilities, a market of money as well as ideas. Investment bank analysts, whose business includes trying to predict the future of both individual companies and the financial markets as a whole, assigned shifting probabilities to the four outcomes through the spring of 2012 (Fig. 14.2).

Before the oral arguments, investment analysts prognosticated a 60 % probability that the entire ACA would be upheld. They thought that the probability of the court's striking the mandate or the mandate plus related provisions was about 30 %. That amounted to a 2-1 bet that the mandate at the heart of the ACA was going to be upheld. The investment analysts assigned quite a low probability—only 5 % in each instance—to either the whole law or the terms of the Medicaid expansion being overturned.

After the oral arguments, the investment analysts, views changed, although they didn't do a complete turnaround. Once the tapes and transcripts of the oral arguments and, even more significant, the justices' questions became available, the

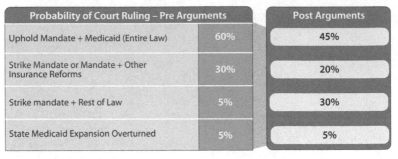

Financial Sector Speculated on ACA Ruling

Investment bank analysts developed probabilities of outcomes around possible SCOTUS rulings pre and post arguments before the Court

Probability of Court Ruling – Pre Arguments		Post Arguments
Uphold Mandate + Medicaid (Entire Law)	60%	45%
Strike Mandate or Mandate + Other Insurance Reforms	30%	20%
Strike mandate + Rest of Law	5%	30%
State Medicaid Expansion Overturned	5%	5%

Fig. 14.2 Confidence in upholding the law decreased after legal arguments were presented to SCOTUS. Source: based on analysis from the Marwood Group Advisory, LLC, 2012

analysts still rated the upholding of the entire law, including the mandate and Medicaid expansion, as the likeliest outcome. But they only assigned upholding the law a 45 % chance of occurring, rather than 60 %.

Analysts lowered their estimate of the Supreme Court's overturning the mandate or mandate plus related provisions to 20 %. But they assigned a much higher probability than before the oral arguments to the possibility that the court would strike down the mandate and the rest of the law, giving this a 30 % chance of occurring versus the earlier prediction of 5 %. Put these together and the smart money, post-oral arguments, was betting that there was about a 50 % chance of the court's overturning either the entire law, the individual mandate, or the mandate plus related provisions.

The one probability the bank analysts left unchanged was the 5 % chance they gave to the Supreme Court's striking down the terms of the Medicaid expansion. However the oral arguments on this issue were felt inside the Beltway to be a very negative event that caught the Administration and Congress off guard.

The analysts' prognostications for the ACA grew bleaker as the annual Supreme Court session neared its end in June 2012, although they never assigned more than a low probability to the court's overturning the terms of the Medicaid expansion.

A similar trend was evident on the website Intrade, where investors can buy shares in the likelihood of various events. By June 11, 2012, 71 % of Intrade investors buying ACA-related shares were betting that the law would be overturned, and conservative economist Tyler Cowen suggested that this might be because of a leak from within the Supreme Court. A week later, 78 % of Intrade investors buying ACA-related shares were betting that the law would fall.

In the midst of these gloomy predictions, perhaps everyone should have remembered the wisdom of Yogi Berra, who famously observed, "Prediction is very hard, especially about the future." Only two weeks before the Supreme Court announced its decision, Justice Ruth Bader Ginsburg dismissed speculations about the ruling

Theories on SCOTUS Majority Abounded

Numerous legal theories on possible ways to achieve a SCOTUS majority circulated, but experts warned that predictions would be difficult, especially when split decisions on the Court are a likely outcome

Oral arguments are not always best indicator of how the Court will rule

Legal Theories on How SCOTUS Could Uphold ACA	
Kennedy Key Vote	Justice Kennedy seen as key swing vote and best hope for upholding ACA
Bush v. Gore	Footnote in case said ruling only applied to this case which gave Justice Kennedy ability to sign on to the narrowest of rulings – could health insurance market be the same?
Roberts Wants Broader Majority	Chief Justice does not want a split decision (5-4) in case with scope/import so would help achieve broader majority to uphold (6-3) most/all of law
If Mandate Goes Then Reforms Too	If Courts strikes mandate, it would be most inclined to take the federal government's arguments to strike community rating and guaranteed issue

Fig. 14.3 Different legal precedents were considered as possible basis for upholding or striking the law and/or key provisions

by telling a conference of the American Constitution Society, "Those who know don't talk. And those who talk don't know." So for those who supported the ACA, there was still hope about the court's final ruling.

At the same time, legal theorists were speculating about how the Supreme Court might find a way to uphold the ACA. Most of this speculation revolved around Justice Anthony Kennedy, who has provided the swing vote on a number of close rulings since he joined the Supreme Court. There was also a speculation that the Supreme Court might leave the ACA standing because of Chief Justice John Roberts's well-known distaste for closely divided rulings on matters of broad significance (Fig. 14.3).

One theory behind the notion that Justice Kennedy might join the Supreme Court's four liberal justices in voting to uphold the ACA drew a line between his voting with the majority in *Bush v. Gore* and the application of the Commerce Clause to the individual mandate. Some theorized a footnote in the 5-4 ruling in *Bush v. Gore* emphasized that the decision only applies in that single instance and should not be taken as a precedent for any subsequent rulings on political elections. A few Supreme Court observers felt that the narrowness of the in *Bush v. Gore* ruling was a crucial factor in Justice Kennedy's voting for it.

Similarly, the same theory went, the Supreme Court might delineate a very narrow basis for upholding the individual mandate in the ACA. Aside from whether the mandate penalty was or was not a tax, the justices had to decide whether Congress had power under the Commerce Clause to assess a penalty for not purchasing health insurance. If Congress can act to compel people to enter into commerce, what is the limiting principle? If you can tell people to buy insurance and penalize them if they don't, can you likewise tell people to buy broccoli and penalize them if they don't?

The narrow-ruling theory went that the market for health insurance is quite different from the market for broccoli. Even a large number of individuals who don't buy broccoli will not have much of an impact on the market for broccoli. However, when large numbers of individuals sit on the sidelines and don't buy health insurance, they do have an impact on the market for health insurance. When large numbers of people don't buy health insurance, they often wait to purchase insurance when they are greasily ill, which increases health insurance premiums and healthcare costs for everybody.

Thus, a *Bush v. Gore*-like footnote might apply to the ruling on the ACA, to the effect that the mandate to engage in commerce by buying health insurance did not apply to any other sort of commerce. On that basis, the proponents of the narrow-ruling theory argued, Justice Kennedy might be persuaded to vote to uphold the ACA.

With regard to Chief Justice John Roberts, the theory was that he would strive to avoid a close decision against a case as significant for the country as *National Federation of Independent Business v. Sebelius.* Constitutional scholars have noted that Chief Justice Roberts has often spoken and written about the desirability of broad majorities in Supreme Court decisions. So it was thought that if Justice Kennedy voted to uphold the ACA on narrow grounds, Chief Justice Roberts might join with him and the four liberal justices to create a 6-3 decision in favor of the law.

Another fairly popular theory for how the Supreme Court could decide on the case held that if the court struck down the individual mandate, a majority of justices might well accept the federal government's severability argument that only the mandate-related provisions for guaranteed issue and community rating should be struck down with it. This would leave in place the rest of the law, including the Medicaid expansion and numerous provisions for healthcare delivery sustain reform.

As it happened, the public prognosticators and theorists were nearly all wrong. In the 5-4 ruling on June 28, 2012, that upheld the ACA, it was Chief Justice John Roberts, not Justice Anthony Kennedy, who provided the swing vote on the grounds that the mandate penalty was constitutional because it was indeed a tax and thus permissible as part of the government's taxing power. Other justices upheld the constitutionality of the mandate on the grounds that the Commerce Clause permitted Congress to enact it. Thus, the court provided a narrow ruling in support of the mandate only because the justices held different views of what constitutional authority Congress held to enact it.

The conservative wing of the court outvoted the four liberal justices by decreeing that the individual mandate was not permissible under the Commerce Clause. But if Chief Justice Roberts had not broken with the conservative wing and also decided that the mandate penalty was a tax, the ACA would not have survived its review by the Supreme Court.

In what some consider the most surprising turn of events, Chief Justice Roberts also joined with Justice Kennedy and the three other conservative justices on the court to overturn the provision that would have allowed the federal government to withhold all federal Medicaid funding to states that did not accept the law's Medicaid coverage expansion. Although the tenor of the oral arguments presaged the Medicaid ruling, the decision was nonetheless stunning because Congress had in the past attached requirements for states or terms for the receipt of federal funds.

The court's Medicaid ruling meant states have the option of turning down the Medicaid coverage expansion in the ACA without fear of losing funding for their pre-ACA program. Some advocates and healthcare stakeholders have feared the ruling would mean many states will choose not to expand coverage, a result that would severely undercut the coverage goal of the ACA. (About half of the ACA coverage expansion was expected to come within Medicaid, according to Congressional Budget Office estimates.) But the court's Medicaid ruling was narrow: it maintained all the other Medicaid provisions of the ACA that held that states would receive federal matching funds for expanded coverage only if they met the terms of the ACA. Thus, states that did not choose to expand would maintain current funding but also reject significant additional federal spending, as much as $930 billion during the next decade, to insure Americans whose income is up to 133 % of the official federal poverty level.

The financial incentives for states to expand medicaid are significant. (The federal government will pay for 100 % of the cost of expansion for three years and phase down its matching rate to states to 90 % over time, compared to a matching rate of 57 % on average for the pre-ACA portion of Medicaid.) In addition, the ACA provides no alternative mechanism for Americans with income at or below federal poverty to obtain federal funds for health coverage other than through Medicaid. Federal subsidies to purchase private health insurance plans from the soon-to-be-created health insurance "exchanges" are less generous than Medicaid and only available to Americans with incomes between 100 % and 400 % of federal poverty. Thus, it is widely expected that over time most states will expand Medicaid per the ACA, despite the court ruling. States that do not take up the ACA Medicaid expansion will leave a significant portion of their uninsured population without coverage, all while their residents' federal tax dollars will be used to fund other states' Medicaid expansions.

Thus the narrow basis for upholding the ACA's individual mandate was that the mandate penalty is a tax by another name. And the outcome that was least expected, the overturning of the terms of the Medicaid expansion, was the one that came to be.

With dust just settling on the Supreme Court's decision, prognosticators immediately turned their eyes to the November 2012 elections. There were still strong forces opposed to the ACA, and if they triumphed in November, they would be in a position to undo the law via legislative repeal or executive action (Fig. 14.4).

In short, the Supreme Court decision was not the only defining moment for the ACA. Rather it was the first act of a two-act play, in which the November elections represented the true dramatic climax. As November approached, there was agreement on all sides that if the Republicans swept the elections, winning the White House and both houses of Congress, repeal of the ACA was virtually guaranteed.

The only elements of the ACA that it was thought the Republicans might preserve were the Medicare cost reductions, or "pay-fors" in Washington speak. Healthcare providers, such as hospitals and physicians, feared this as the worst of all possible worlds, with money being pulled out of the existing system and no expansion of funding through an expansion of coverage.

November 2012 Elections Tested
Fate of ACA After SCOTUS Ruling

Presidential Election Outcome	Congressional Election Outcome	Possible SCOTUS Decision			Possible Impact on ACA
		Eliminate Entire Law	Eliminate Individual Mandate	Uphold Law	
Romney	Republicans Take Senate and House	✔			Focus turns to deficit & Republican healthcare priorities, i.e., health savings accounts, high risk pools, malpractice
			✔		Repeal coverage expansion, Medicare pay-fors remain
				✔	Repeal coverage expansion, Medicare pay-fors remain
Romney	Democrats Retain Senate	✔			Focus turns to deficit, including Medicare & Medicaid reform
			✔		Possible gridlock, i.e., negotiation on alternatives to mandate do not result in other fixes to ACA
				✔	ACA likely maintained in large form
Obama	Republicans Take Senate and House	✔			Focus turns to deficit reduction, including Medicare & Medicaid reform; marginal insurance market reforms reinstated
			✔		Negotiations on alternatives to mandate result in fixes to ACA
				✔	ACA maintained with possibility for some fixes to be negotiated
Obama	Democrats Retain Senate	✔			Replacement of insurance market reforms, including exchanges
			✔		Replace individual mandate with alternative
				✔	ACA maintained

Fig. 14.4 The ACA was again publicly debated during the 2012 election campaign. The law was in danger of repeal should the Republicans win the Presidency and/or majority seats in the US Senate and US House of Representatives. (Source: based on analysis from the Marwood Group Advisory, LLC, 2012)

If the Democrats swept the election, maintaining control of the Senate and giving President Obama a second term, then obviously the law would remain intact and its implementation would proceed.

With divided government (where Republicans and Democrats split control of the legislative and executive branches), the ACA would also likely remain in place. Divided government of any kind would almost certainly keep the Republicans from repealing the law, although it might result in modifications of greater or lesser importance if a Republican was elected to the White House.

The perceived closeness of the approaching elections gave impetus to the same intensity of speculation about the ACA's ultimate fate as there was on the eve of the Supreme Court decision. Many factors seemed to point to divided government as the most likely scenario after November 2012. On the one hand, President Obama retained an edge over Mitt Romney in polling through the summer, On the other hand, the Democrats faced difficulties in maintaining their slim majority in the Senate, owing to the fact that they had many more seats up in 2012 than the Republicans (Fig. 14.5). The Democrats had 21 Senate seats in play, 23 counting the two seats of the Independent senators who caucused with them, whereas the Republicans had only 10 Senate seats in play and fewer seats to defend. With numbers like these, control of the Senate seemed destined to change hands in 2012.

The results of the November elections maintained divided government at the federal level, even though the results favored Democrats overall (Democrats had a net *gain* of two seats in the Senate and 13 seats in the House). The reasons for these

2012 Elections In Congress Favored Republicans But Democrats Retained Senate

• Number of open seats and retirements favored Republicans in both Senate and House races in 2012, but Democrates retained majority in Senate

• Majority in Senate better enables Democrats to protect ACA from setbacks

Senate Race (60 seats for super majority)				House Race (218 seats for majority)		
	Seats (prior to election)	Open Seats in 2012			112th Congress (Prior to election)	Retirements
Democratic Seats	51 +2 independent	21 +2 independent	9 of which have historically favored Republicans (MT, NM, ND, NE, MO, OH, FL, VA, WV)	Republican Seats	242	10
Republican Seats	47	10	2 of which have historically favored Democrats (ME, MA)	Democratic Seats	193	15
Total	100	33		Total	435	25

Fig. 14.5 The outcome of 2012 election would determine major fiscal and healthcare policies. (Source: based on analysis from the Marwood Group Advisory, LLC, 2012)

results are numerous and have been the subject of much reflection within both political parties. Suffice it to say they reflect the net effect of both the successes earned by winning candidates and the missteps made by losing candidates. Moreover, the election results sealed the Supreme Court's ruling over the ACA as the law of the land and set back its critics for at least two years and possibly four. President Obama will have a window of time to in which he can implement the ACA and make it part of the fabric of America's healthcare system before another round of political gamesmanship is at hand in 2014 and 2016.

When Congress undertakes major policy innovation, the fate of a law remains uncertain as in the case of the ACA. Major laws can be challenged in court. Even when a court decision is handed down, it could have uncertain outcomes as was the case with the Supreme Court's decision on the ACA Medicaid expansion. Major laws can be viewed as unwelcome by the public and repealed, as was the case with the Medicare Catastrophic Coverage Act of 1988. Although not every year, Congress proceeds in passing major policy innovations despite these types of uncertainties because its members learn quickly that there is no perfect law. Legislation is almost always imperfect—especially major policy innovations—and modified at a minimum to fix drafting errors and address issues that were not foreseen. Thus, Congress does not usually intend new policy innovations to be static. The challenge with a controversial law such as the ACA is that continued opposition will hamper Congress' ability to aptly fine-tune the law through future legislation. Thus, the next phase of modifications to the ACA experiment will come through the regulatory process, except in rare cases where Congress and the President will be able to agree to make changes.

Arguably, the polarized political dynamics surrounding passage of the ACA sowed the seeds of opposition that led to the Supreme Court challenges and numerous calls for repeal from Republican candidates during the November elections. Could Democrats and Republicans have come to agreement on a less controversial version of the law? Many have asserted that the 111th Congress could have passed a bipartisan bill that would have avoided substantial judicial and political challenge. However, history tells otherwise. Landmark pieces of healthcare legislation, such as the law creating Medicare and Medicaid, were similarly polarized before, during, and after passage.

In the case of the ACA, the Chairman of the Senate Finance Committee, Senator Max Baucus (D-MT), tried valiantly to negotiate a bipartisan compromise on the ACA, but to no avail. The Senate version of the ACA passed the chamber on December 24, 2009, with a strict party-line vote. Congress had been deeply divided over expanding health insurance coverage not just during passage of ACA but for over 100 years leading up to it. Attempts to pass universal health reform failed acrimoniously several times during the twentieth century. Hence, the polarization surrounding the ACA is part of the long history of debate over establishing universal access to health insurance coverage in the US.

Chapter 15
Medicaid Expansion Challenges States

JudyAnn Bigby

Twenty-six states joined the suit to stop the Affordable Care Act, in part because of the requirement that states expand Medicaid eligibility for adults or give up participating in the program entirely. The Supreme Court ruling restricted Congress' authority to amend the terms under which states participate in the Medicaid program. The decision was surprising to some because in the past Congress has amended the Medicaid law to require states to expand coverage to certain populations including poor pregnant women and children [1]. As a result of the ruling, states may continue their state Medicaid program without expanding eligibility as defined by the ACA. However, they are required to maintain the eligibility standards that were in place on March 23, 2010, when the ACA was enacted. States must maintain adult eligibility standards until health insurance exchanges are certified and child eligibility standards until 2019. States may expand coverage to low-income, nonelderly adults. Through this option Medicaid remains an important mechanism for states to insure more Americans, especially poor adults. According to Jost and Rosenbaum [1], Chief Justice Roberts acknowledged that "under the ACA Medicaid had become an important element in a comprehensive plan to achieve universal health insurance coverage in the U.S."

Contrary to many people's assumption that Medicaid provides health coverage for "poor" people, federal law prior to passage of the ACA mandated eligibility only for pregnant women and children under age six with family incomes at or below 133 % FPL, children ages 6–18 with family incomes at or below 100 % FPL, parents and caretaker relatives who meet the financial eligibility requirements for the former Aid to Families with Dependent Children cash assistance (welfare) program, and blind, elderly, and disabled people who qualify for Supplemental Security

J. Bigby, M.D. (✉)
Formerly Health and Human Services, Boston, MA, USA
e-mail: Judy.bigby@comcast.net

H.P. Selker and J.S. Wasser (eds.), *The Affordable Care Act as a National Experiment:*
Health Policy Innovations and Lessons, DOI 10.1007/978-1-4614-8351-9_15,
© Springer Science+Business Media New York 2014

Income benefits based on low income and resources. Federal law prior to the ACA excluded nondisabled, nonpregnant adults without dependent children, unless states used the Medicaid 1115 demonstration waiver program to make them eligible. The ACA Medicaid eligibility expansion, therefore, particularly benefits childless adults and low-income parents who may not qualify for Medicaid even if their children qualify. The ACA expands the Medicaid program's mandatory coverage groups by requiring that participating states cover nearly all people under age 65 with household incomes at or below 133 % FPL ($15,282 per year for an individual and $32,322 per year for a family of four in 2013) beginning in January, 2014 (Table 15.1). Because there is an allowance to disregard up to 5 % of income, the effective eligibility level is up to 138 % FPL.

Table 15.1 Medicaid eligibility categories and income thresholds before and after the ACA

Categorical groups	US minimum income threshold before ACA, 2009	State actual median income thresholds, 2009 (ranges)	Categorical groups after ACA	US proposed minimum income thresholds under ACA, 2014
Children 0–5	133 % FPL[a]	235 % FPL (133–300 % FPL)	Children (ages 0–18 years)	133 % FPL
Children 6–19	100 % FPL	235 % FPL (100–300 % FPL)		
Pregnant women	133 % FPL	185 % FPL (133–300 % FPL)	Adults (ages 19–64 years)	133 % FPL
Working parents	State's July 1996 TANF[b] eligibility level	64 % FPL (17–200 % FPL)		
Nonworking parents	State's July 1996 TANF eligibility level	38 % FPL (11–200 % FPL)		
Childless adults	Eligibility not mandated. May cover with waiver	0 % FPL (0 % FPL in 46 states; 100–160 % FPL in 5 states)		
Elderly, blind, disabled	Receipt of supplemental security income	75 % FPL (65–133 % FPL)	Elderly, blind, disabled	Receipt of supplemental security income

(Source: Musumeci M, Artiga S, Rudowitz R. Medicaid eligibility, simplification, and coordination under the Affordable Care Act: A summary of CMS's August 17, 2011, proposed rule and key issues to be considered. Kaiser Commission on Medicaid and the Uninsured. Henry Kaiser Family Foundation. October 2011)

Categorical groups must meet certain citizen requirements

In states that choose to expand Medicaid, the threshold will be at or above the new US minimum threshold starting in 2014. If a state's threshold was already higher, states may maintain the higher threshold

[a]Federal poverty level

[b]Temporary assistance to needy families

To Expand or Not to Expand?

As a result of the Supreme Court ruling, it is up to the individual states whether or not they agree to expand Medicaid eligibility and they no longer need to worry about jeopardizing their current Medicaid funding. As the January 2014 start date for expanding Medicaid eligibility approaches and state legislative sessions during which most states need to enact laws or modify their budgets to authorize expansion conclude, there have been intense debates about whether and how to expand. There is great diversity of opinion and strong emotional arguments not only between states but also among decision makers in states. Business leaders, hospitals and other providers, and healthcare advocates have weighed in with their opinions in state houses, opinion pages, and anywhere else they think they can be heard.

States share the cost of the Medicaid program with the federal government at varying levels, with some states paying less than 50 % of the costs. The ACA mandates that the federal government pick up most of the costs to cover the populations covered by the eligibility expansion. For most states, the federal government will cover 100 % of the states' costs of the coverage expansion from 2014 to 2016, gradually decreasing to 90 % in 2020 and subsequent years. States that expanded eligibility prior to passage of the ACA will also receive an increase in the federal contribution for the expansion populations but initial rates start at 75 % (Table 15.2). The ACA also requires the benefit package for the newly eligible Medicaid populations meet the definition of "essential health benefits," thus preventing states from offering less comprehensive coverage to the newly eligible populations.

States that will likely expand eligibility, As of March 2013, sixteen states (CA, CO, CT, DE, HI, MA, MD, MN, NM, NJ, NV, NY, OR, RI, VT, WA) and the District of Columbia will expand Medicaid eligibility and have already taken the necessary steps to participate. Hawaii, Massachusetts, and Vermont represent three of the four states that expanded eligibility prior to the ACA. Three of the states (New Jersey, New Mexico, and Nevada) have Republican governors who now support expansion and appear to have the backing of their state legislatures. Colorado, Nevada, and Washington were among the plaintiff states.

The arguments for expanding Medicaid eligibility in the states are diverse. Business leaders, healthcare providers, nonprofits, patient advocates, city and

Table 15.2 Federal share of cost of Medicaid eligibility expansion, 2014–2020 and beyond

Year	States without expanded eligibility (%)	States with expanded eligibility prior to ACA (%)
2014	100	75
2015	100	80
2016	100	85
2017	95	86
2018	94	89.6
2019	93	93
2020 and beyond	90	90

county governments, and others have joined forces to focus on the benefits of expansion including the increased revenue that states will gain, the impact on providers who serve the uninsured, the impact on the health of the expansion populations, the lack of other options for individuals who even with subsidies will not be able to afford exchange products or won't have access to the exchange, and the economic impact on states. Recent reports document the impact of Medicaid coverage on mortality reduction [2] and on increasing access to necessary care [3].

States that are not likely to expand eligibility, As of March 2013, ten states (AK, AL, GA, ID, LA, MS, NC, OK, SC, and TX) are not likely to expand their eligibility for adults to participate in Medicaid. Alabama Governor Bently indicated that he would not expand Medicaid as it currently exists and wants to reform the program before considering expansion. Government officials in North Carolina and other states cite the need to better manage the Medicaid program before expanding. State legislatures have generally supported the governors' decisions not to expand eligibility in these states. However in some circumstances the minority Democratic Party, business leaders, healthcare advocates, and others have lobbied for expansion arguing that federal revenue supporting expansion will stimulate the states' economy and help healthcare providers get through difficult financial challenges. Hospitals in these states are especially concerned as Disproportionate Share Hospital spending will decline as required in the ACA. Texas Governor Rick Perry (R) has maintained his position opposing expansion even in light of strong lobbying from the Chamber of Commerce and hospitals [4].

The states that are unlikely to expand have some of the lowest income eligibility thresholds for adults and have high rates of uninsured. These states also have the largest populations of individuals who delay needed medical care. Counties in states with eligibility criteria set below 133 % FPL have a disproportionately higher percent of populations reporting they delay needed care because of costs [5]. These states must provide medical assistance for children and adults who are eligible under the pre-ACA standards at the standard level of federal match (Table 15.3). While these states and their residents have the most to gain in terms of decreasing the percent of uninsured and improving access to care, they also will have the largest costs.

States that have resisted Medicaid expansion cite other reasons not to expand including their desire to repeal the ACA entirely, the cost to the state, the cost to the federal government, people dropping private insurance and opting for Medicaid coverage (crowd out), concern that the federal share will decrease below the 90 % required in the ACA after 2020 (or sooner!), the uncertainty of the impact of proposed cuts to Medicare and Medicaid, the lack of providers to care for the population, and the access to insurance that some low-income individuals will have in the exchange.

The experience in Massachusetts and other states that have already expanded Medicaid eligibility provides some insight into the level of validity of some of these concerns. For example, crowd out of private insurance did not occur and the percentage of employers offering insurance increased after Massachusetts implemented the 2006 reform law [6]. In spite of widespread reports about the lack of primary care providers, more people reported they had a regular source of care after reform [7].

Table 15.3 States' positions on expanding Medicaid[a], the status of eligibility thresholds, uninsured, and federal funding

	Medicaid benefits eligibility (% FPL) without ACA		Rate of uninsurance among adult population <65 years old ≤133 % FPL	Projected incremental number covered with expanded eligibility (thousands)[b]	Percent of Medicaid budget that is federal prior to ACA
	Parents (unemployed/ employed)	Childless (unemployed/ employed)			
States not likely to expand					
Alabama[c]	10/23	n/a	41	313	68.5
Alaska[c]	74/78	n/a	34	37	50
Georgia[c]	27/48	n/a	49	698	65.56
Idaho[c]	20/37	n/a	35	88	71
Louisiana[c]	11/24	n/a	50	398	61.24
Mississippi[c]	23/29	n/a	46	231	73.43
North Carolina	34/47	n/a	33	568	65.51
Oklahoma	36/51	n/a	32	204	64
South Carolina[c]	50/89	n/a	38	312	70.43
Texas[c]	12/25	n/a	43	1,805	59.3
States undecided[d]					
Arizona[c]	100/106	100	40	238	65.68
Arkansas	13/16	n/a			70.17
Florida[c]	19/56	n/a	53	1,276	58.08
Illinois	133–139	n/a	44	573	50
Indiana[c]	18/24	n/a	35	495	67.16
Iowa[e]	27/80	n/a	36	72	59.59
Kansas[c]	25/31	n/a	29	169	56.51
Kentucky	33/57	n/a	41	268	70.55
Maine[c]	200/200	n/a	25	45	62.57
Michigan[c]	37/64	n/a	38	345	66.39
Missouri	18/35	n/a	40	383	61.37

(continued)

Table 15.3 (continued)

	Medicaid benefits eligibility (% FPL) without ACA		Rate of uninsurance among adult population <65 years old ≤133 % FPL	Projected incremental number covered with expanded eligibility (thousands)[b]	Percent of Medicaid budget that is federal prior to ACA
	Parents (unemployed/ employed)	Childless (unemployed/ employed)			
Montana	31/54	n/a	50	64	66
Nebraska[c]	47/58	n/a	38	88	55.76
New Hampshire	38/47	n/a	37	42	50
North Dakota[c]	33/57	n/a	39	32	52.27
Ohio[c]	90/96	n/a	47	684	63.58
Pennsylvania[c]	25/58	n/a	32	542	54.28
South Dakota[c]	50/50	n/a	42	44	56.19
Tennessee	67/122	n/a	39	363	66.13
Utah[c]	37/42	n/a	38	189	68.61
Virginia[c]	25/30	n/a	43	327	50
West Virginia	16/31	n/a	36	116	72.04
Wisconsin[c]	200/200	n/a	33	211	59.74
Wyoming[c]	37/50	n/a	47	27	50
States likely to expand					
California	100/106	n/a	46	1,860	50
Connecticut	185/191	55/70	30	150	50
Colorado[c]	100/106	10/20 (closed)	44	225	50
Delaware	100/120	100/110	29	16	55.67
Hawaii	133/133	133/133	23	62	51.86
Maryland	116/122	n/a	37	146	50
Massachusetts	133	300	12	16	50
Minnesota	215/215	75/75	31	105	50
Nevada[c]	24/84	n/a	53	137	59.74

New Jersey	200/200 (closed for >133 %)	n/a	44	291	50
New Mexico	28/85	n/a	46	208	69.07
New York	150/150	100/100	31	320	50
Oregon	30/39	n/a	41	400	62.44
Rhode Island	175/181	n/a	36	40	51.26
Vermont	185/191	150/160	22	3	56.04
Washington[e]	35/71	n/a	41	137	50

(Sources: [a]State Activity Around Expanding Medicaid Under the Affordable Care Act. http://www.StateHealthFacts.org [Accessed March 5, 2013] Status of the ACA Medicaid Expansion after Supreme Court Ruling. Center on Budget and Policy. March 13, 2013
[b]Holahan J et al. The Cost and Coverage Implications of the ACA Medicaid Expansion: National and State-by-State Analysis. Kaiser Commission for Medicaid and the Uninsured. Henry J Kaiser Family Foundation. November 2012)
[c]Plaintiff states who challenged the constitutionality of ACA
[d]States still analyzing their options, in conversations with HHS, and/or legislature and governor in disagreement
[e]Iowa and Washington were on both sides of the case, as their governors and attorneys general took opposite positions

Some states have argued that the population is difficult to care for and they do not have the appropriate resources to provide care. However, the demographics of the expansion population are similar to the currently eligible population except for the higher percent of males. More than half the population is under 35 years old and 13 % are between the ages of 55 and 64. Fifty-three percent of the uninsured who would be newly eligible for Medicaid are male. The majority (55 %) is white, 19 % are Hispanic, 19 % are black, and 7 % are in the "other race" category. More than 90 % of the newly eligible are citizens. More than half of the population is employed. The population has a history of frequent emergency department use and may have significant behavioral health problems [8].

The Next Battleground: State Legislatures and Governor Offices—The remainder of the states have either not made final decisions about expanding Medicaid eligibility or there is disagreement between the governors and legislative bodies on whether to expand. Several states are still analyzing the advantages and risks of participating. Among these states (Table 15.3) the Urban Institutes estimates that for some states the cost of expanding eligibility with the enhanced federal contribution would be cost neutral or result in savings (Iowa, Maine, New Hampshire, and Wisconsin) or result in less than a two percent increase in state costs (Arizona, Illinois, Minnesota, Nebraska) [9].

Many of the plaintiff states declared that they would not participate in expanding Medicaid eligibility soon after the Supreme Court ruling. Governor Rick Scott (R) of Florida and Governor Jan Brewer (R) of Arizona sent shock waves across the country when they announced their intention to participate. Governor Brewer filed legislation that recommends expanding eligibility, using Medicaid managed care plans. Governor Scott proposed enrolling the expansion population in private insurance plans when he announced his plan to expand eligibility [10]. The Arizona and Florida legislatures have not endorsed their governors' plans thus far [11]. One Republican leader referred to Governor Brewer as "Judas" because of her support. However patients, business leaders, healthcare officials, supporters of AARP, and more than 100 other organizations have backed Governor Brewer's plan [12]. Governor Scott's plan was blocked in the legislature. The Florida legislature is instead exploring other ways to develop a "not-Medicaid plan" for those who would be newly covered [13].

Other states have considered a middle ground approach to expanding eligibility which they believe is more acceptable than expanding the state Medicaid program. Arkansas Governor Mike Beebe (D) announced an agreement with HHS to use the federal enhanced revenue to purchase insurance for the expansion population through the exchange even though the cost of insurance in the exchange could be more expensive than Medicaid coverage [14]. The secretary of HHS has apparently demonstrated a willingness to be flexible about how states implement the expanded eligibility. But Tennessee Governor Bill Haslam (R) announced that his state would not expand Medicaid because the administration put too many conditions on how the state could use the money [15]. Governor Branstad (R) of Iowa wants to improve IowaCare, a program that serves as a safety net for low-income populations. The program would focus on preventive healthcare and help people to stay healthy.

However the current program offers very minimal coverage [16]. Wisconsin Governor Scott Walker (R) announced his rejection of the Medicaid expansion and proposed an alternative plan that would cover low-income adults through purchase of private insurance in the federally operated exchange [17]. Wisconsin democrats are not satisfied that they have sufficient detail about this plan. Some may view Wisconsin's proposed reliance on the federal exchange as ironic since some states that opposed the ACA have requested that the federal government give them more flexibility to design programs that meet their states' population needs.

Some states are also identifying ways to mitigate some of the potential risks of participation as a condition of their participation. For example, some states have included statutory language in authorizing legislation or in budget language that allows them to abandon expanding eligibility if the federal share of the cost of expansion decreases substantially below 90 %. Arizona has proposed to fund the state share of the cost using a provider assessment to generate the necessary revenue.

Many states have engaged independent consultants to analyze the advantages and risks in expanding eligibility [19]. Governor Gary Herbert (R) of Utah indicated he will make a final decision about expansion only after a state-commissioned study by the Public Consulting Group is complete and resisted pressure from state democrats to accelerate the timeline. States are also analyzing the economic impact of expanded eligibility on the states. For example, Governor Brewer used the analysis by the Grand Canyon Institute that concluded that fully implementing the ACA would add 21,000 new jobs and increase economic growth by $2.776 billion or 0.6 % [20] to bolster her recommendation to expand.

Maine is in a unique situation, as an early expansion state, where the governor resisted expansion while the legislature supports expansion. As an early expansion state, in January 2014, Maine may replace current state spending to cover the expansion populations with federal dollars as set forth in the ACA. After initially rejecting the possibility of expansion, Governor LePage has reconsidered and has asked the Secretary of Health and Human Services to pay the entire cost of covering the expansion population for 10 years [18].

Time is money—The Centers for Medicare and Medicaid Services (CMS) has stated that there is no deadline by which states must decide whether to expand or not. However, the 100 % federal match is only available to states in the years of the expansion as set forth in the ACA to cover costs associated with the pent up demand for health services by the expansion population. The ACA enables the enhanced federal match at 100 % through 2016 and sets forth a schedule for decreasing the match to 90 % by 2020. According to communications from the Department of Health and Human Services, the law does not provide for a phased-in or partial expansion [21].

Implementing the ACA is an ongoing endeavor. As of July 2013, there had been considerable movement in states' plans to expand Medicaid. Only six states - MI, IN, OH, PA, NH, and TN - were still debating whether to expand. Twenty-one states were not moving forward with a January 2014 expansion. Twenty-four states including the District of Colombia were moving forward (http://kff.org/medicaid/issue-brief/analyzing-the-impact-of-state-medicaid-expansion-decisions).

Potential Impact of Expanded Medicaid Eligibility
on Uninsurance Rates

The Urban Institute conducted an analysis that estimates that if all states participate in expanding eligibility for Medicaid, 21.3 million additional people would enroll in Medicaid by 2022 [9]. Some of the enrollees would be newly eligible under the ACA rules, but a significant proportion would be individuals that states have had the option of covering. Even if states do not elect to participate in the Medicaid eligibility expansion, the Congressional Budget Office (CBO) estimates that all states will experience growth in the numbers who are insured by the Medicaid program [22]. Individuals will seek out or become aware of their eligibility for Medicaid as allowed by pre-ACA rules because of pressure arising from the individual mandate and widespread public education about options for coverage. The ACA also provides for a streamlined enrollment and eligibility process which will make it easier for those who are already eligible to enroll [23]. In addition, those seeking to purchase insurance in the exchange will automatically be screened for Medicaid eligibility.

Some of the individuals who would have been eligible for Medicaid under the expanded eligibility rules will still have access to insurance coverage. Individuals with incomes between 100 % and 138 % of the FPL will be eligible to purchase insurance through the exchange with federal subsidies to defray the cost premium and out-of-pocket cost sharing. Even though some low-income individuals will find it burdensome to pay even a small part of the premium to take advantage of this coverage, some are likely to find a way to purchase coverage in the exchange. In addition, more children who are currently eligible for Medicaid or CHIP may end up being enrolled because parents cannot purchase insurance through the exchange unless their children are covered.

The CBO estimates that by 2022 the number of individuals purchasing insurance in the exchange will increase from 22 million to 25 million as a result of the Supreme Court ruling and that the number enrolling in CHIP and Medicaid will decrease from their original estimate of 17 million to 11 million.[1] The overall decrease in the number of insured was revised down to 30 million from 33 million [22].

Because the ACA provides federal tax credits to individuals and families to purchase insurance in the exchange only if their incomes are between 100 % and 400 % FPL, populations with incomes below 100 % FPL will continue to have difficulty accessing affordable health insurance in states that decide not to participate in expansion of Medicaid eligibility. Individuals at this income level are not eligible to receive federal subsidies to purchase insurance in the exchange. They are unlikely to be able to find affordable, unsubsidized health insurance. Legal immigrants are an exception as they are eligible to purchase in the exchange with incomes at 0–400 % FPL.

---

[1] Note that the estimates by the Urban Institute and the Congressional Budget Office for the newly enrolled Medicaid populations differ.

Potential Impact of the ACA and Expanded Medicaid Eligibility on State and Federal Spending

State spending—The projected cost to state Medicaid programs as a result of the ACA stems from two scenarios. First, even without participating in the expanded Medicaid eligibility, they will see their state Medicaid enrollment (as discussed above) and associated costs increase. If states participate in the Medicaid eligibility expansion, there are additional costs associated with that population. The Urban Institute estimates that if all states expand Medicaid eligibility, the total costs for covering both the already eligible and the expansion populations would be $76 billion [8] (Figs. 15.1 and 15.2). The Urban Institute estimates that $68 billion in costs are attributable to the take up of Medicaid by the already eligible populations. The incremental state cost of implementing Medicaid expansion would be only $8 billion for the period 2013–2022. The incremental cost of expansion represents a 0.3 % increase in state spending under the ACA compared to the costs of implementing the ACA without expansion.

Between 2014 and 2019, several states (Hawaii, Maine, Massachusetts, and Vermont) that have already expanded eligibility could save state dollars because the federal government would pay an increased share of the cost of covering the expanded eligibility population. Massachusetts Governor Deval Patrick's proposed FY14 state budget estimates that implementing the ACA Medicaid expansion will generate $175.5 million in enhanced federal revenue because the federal share of the cost of Medicaid for the expansion populations increases from 50 % to 75 % in FY14. The state estimates they would spend only $25.8 million to cover individuals who are not already enrolled under the state's existing Medicaid expansion. The net savings is therefore approximately $150 million (see "Expanding Access to Affordable Quality Healthcare, FY14 Budget Recommendations, Issues in Brief." http://www.mass.gov/bb/h1/fy14h1/exec_14/hbudbrief3.htm).

States that would require substantially increased state spending (4–7 % over current state spending) under ACA if they expand eligibility are largely those from the South and they cap eligibility at the lowest income thresholds [9]. Even though these states receive the highest share of federal contribution (59–73 %), they are worried about the impact on their state budgets. They would spend the most to cover the populations that are already eligible for Medicaid before benefiting from the increased federal revenue for covering the expansion populations (see Table 15.3).

Several analyses demonstrate that in addition to generating more federal revenue for their Medicaid programs, states would achieve significant state budget savings resulting from expanding Medicaid eligibility and enrolling those individuals in Medicaid. Many states currently use state-only money for programs to provide categorical services for the uninsured and do not receive matching federal revenue for providing these services. These programs include uncompensated care, prescription drug programs for the underinsured and uninsured, outpatient and inpatient mental health services, health coverage for children in foster care and youth who age out of foster care, and cancer, HIV, and other disease-specific programs. Some of the

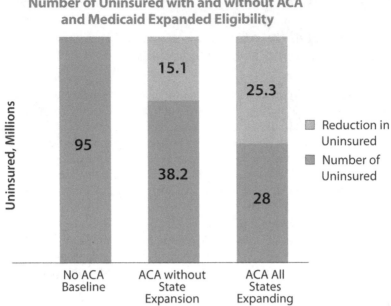

Fig. 15.1 State expansion of Medicaid covers a greater number of individuals. Reproduced with permission from Holahan J, et al. Cost and Coverage Implications of the ACA Medicaid Expansion: National and State-by-State Analysis. Kaiser Commission on Medicaid and the Uninsured. November, 2012. Kaiser Family Foundation, 2012

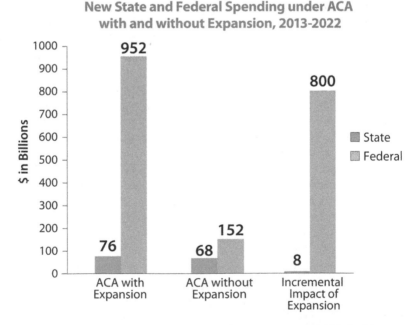

Fig. 15.2 It will cost the Federal and State governments more to expand Medicaid coverage by 2022. Reproduced with permission from Holahan J, et al. Cost and Coverage Implications of the ACA Medicaid Expansion: National and State-by-State Analysis. Kaiser Commission on Medicaid and the Uninsured. November, 2012. Kaiser Family Foundation, 2012

populations who use these services will become insured and have access to comprehensive coverage under the ACA provisions, and states will either receive federal revenue to replace a portion of the state dollars or be able to avoid state spending altogether if individuals are eligible to purchase insurance in the exchange. States will save an estimated $18 billion in non-Medicaid costs on these types of programs. If all states expand Medicaid eligibility, states overall will see a net savings of $10 billion [9]. Additional financial benefits to states are projected due to additional impact the expansion may have on access to certain medical care [22].

Federal spending—If all states choose to expand Medicaid eligibility, between 2013 and 2022, federal spending would increase by $952 billion. Even if states do not expand Medicaid eligibility, federal spending on Medicaid would increase by $152 billion due to increases in Medicaid enrollment under existing Medicaid eligibility rules (as discussed above). Therefore $800 billion of the $952 billion in increased spending is due to the expansion of Medicaid eligibility and the federal government bearing the bulk of the cost of expansion [9].

In addition, the CBO estimates that as a result of the Supreme Court ruling, federal spending on the ACA will decrease by $84 billion from the original CBO estimate. In states where eligibility for Medicaid is not expanded, more individuals with incomes between 100 % and 138 % of FPL would use federal subsidies to purchase insurance and to decrease cost sharing in the exchange. The CBO estimates that about half of the people who would have obtained Medicaid coverage through expanded eligibility will use the exchange to purchase insurance with federal subsidies. The reduction in spending from lower Medicaid enrollment more than offsets the increase in costs associated with greater participation in the exchange [22].

Conclusion

The ACA, while a promising vehicle for expanding access to insurance and healthcare, is also controversial. Some states have been philosophically opposed to using government to provide health insurance or have been concerned about the size of the Medicaid program and its impact on state budgets. When the Medicaid program was first passed in 1965, states made some of the same arguments for and against participating in the new program as they have offered about participating in expanding Medicaid eligibility. States were leery of the costs to their budgets but at the same time saw the potential to receive federal support for some programs they were already offering. There was wide variation in the way states implemented the original Medicaid program. By 1967, 22 states enlarged their programs to deliver healthcare to the poor. By 1969 all but two states, Arizona and Alaska, committed to the Medicaid program [24]. Arizona was the last state to participate and designed a unique program with approval by Department of Health and Human Services. History suggests that states may find a way to take advantage of the ACA to improve healthcare access for residents of their states. While all states may not agree to participate in expanded Medicaid eligibility beginning in January 2014, the ACA is a good foundation for enabling states to eventually figure out a way to participate and offer coverage to the millions of uninsured who would benefit. Historically, the federal government has allowed flexibility in how states design their Medicaid programs. There are 50 different state programs across the USA. Clearly the federal government does not believe "one size fits all."

The ACA offers a real opportunity to decrease the number of uninsured Americans. It is unfortunate that the opportunity for states to expand eligibility for Medicaid comes at a time when state budgets are still reeling from the recession and there is uncertainty about federal budget cuts. The legitimate concerns of states about the costs and about the need to improve the Medicaid program emphasize the need to reform the delivery system and eliminate wasteful healthcare spending. Fortunately, the ACA offers tremendous opportunities to advance this agenda as well. States should consider both opportunities as they weigh the decision to participate fully in the Medicaid expansion.

References

1. Jost TS, Rosenbaum S. The supreme court and the future of medicaid. N Engl J Med. 2012;367:983–5.
2. Sommers BD, Baicker K, Epstein AM. Mortality and access to care among adults after state medicaid expansions. N Engl J Med. 2012;367:1025–34.
3. Baicker K, Finkelstein A. The effects of medicaid coverage—learning from the Oregon experiment. N Engl J Med. 2011;365:683–5.
4. Fernandez M. Texans rebut Governor Rick Perry on expansion of Medicaid. New York Times. 2013; March 4.
5. Clark CR, Ommerborn MJ, Coull BA, Pham DQ. H J. State Medicaid eligibility and care delayed because of cost. N Engl J Med. 2013;368:1263–5.
6. Long SK, Stockley K. Employer coverage from employees' perspective. Health Aff. 2009;28: 1079–87.
7. Long SK, Masi PB. Access and affordability: an update on health reform in Massachusetts, Fall 2008. Health Aff. 2009;28:w578–87.
8. Kenney GM, Zuckerman S, Dubay L, Huntress M, Lynch V, Haley J, Anderson N. Opting in to the medicaid expansion under the ACA: who are the uninsured adults who could gain health insurance coverage? Urban Institute August 2012. http://www.urban.org/UploadedPDF/412630-opting-in-medicaid.pdf.
9. Holahan J, Buettgens M, Carroll C, Dorn S. The cost and coverage implications of the ACA medicaid expansion: national and state-by-state analysis. Kaiser Commission for Medicaid and the Uninsured. Henry J Kaiser Family Foundation. Nov 2012.
10. Krugman P. Mooching off medicaid. http://www.nytimes.com/2013/03/04/opinion/krugman-mooching-off-medicare.html?_r=0 New York Times. 3 Mar 2013.
11. Reinhart MK. Brewer unveils legislation to broaden Medicaid eligibility. Governor's plan includes olive branch to GOP legislators. 2013; March 13. Also: Alvarez L. Medicaid expansion is rejected in Florida. New York Times. 2013; March 11.
12. Reinhart MK. Republicans split on Medicaid expansion. 2013; March 23. Available from: http://www.azcentral.com/news/politics/articles/2013032republican-medicaid-expansion.html.
13. Gentry C. In Florida, Medicaid expansion may be dead, but expanding coverage isn't, Health News Florida. 2013; Mar 14. Available from: http://www.kaiserhealthnews.org/stories/2013/march/14/ medicaid-expansion-plan-florida.aspx.

14. Goodnough A. Governor of Tennessee joins peers refusing Medicaid plan. 2013; March 27. Available from: http://www.nytimes.com/2013/03/28/health/tennessee-governor-balks-at-medicaid-expansion. html?_r=0.
15. Lucey C. Branstad keeps focus on IowaCare, not Medicaid. The Atlanta Journal-Constitution 2013; March 3.
16. Spicuzza M. Scott Walker rejects Medicaid expansion, proposes alternate plan to cover uninsured. Wisconsin State Journal. 2013. Feb 14, Available from: http://host.madison.com/wsj/news/local/govtand-politics/on-politics/on-politics-gov-scott-walker-announces-he-is-rejecting-federal/article_3bf0f724-7617-11e2-b2aa-0019bb2963f4.html.
17. Roy A. Arkansas: replacing medicaid expansion with Obamacare's exchanges could require 'no additional federal costs at all'. http://www.forbes.com/sites/aroy/2013/03/19/arkansas-replacing-medicaid-expansion-with-obamacares-exchanges-could-require-no-additional-federal-costs-at-all/. Forbes. 19 March 2013.
18. Mistler S. Maine Hospital Association backs Medicaid expansion. Portland Press Herald. 2013; March 28.
19. http://www.familiesusa.org/issues/medicaid/expansion-center/resources-from-the-states.html.
20. Wells D. Arizona's medicaid options under the affordable care act: fiscal and economic consequences. Grand Canyon Institute. Sept 2012. https://grandcanyoninstitute.org/sites/grandcanyoninstitute.org/files/GCI_Policy_Arizona_Medicaid_Options_Sept_2012.pdf.
21. Secretary Sebelius letter to Governors. 12 Dec 2012. http://www.cciio.cms.gov/resources/files/gov-letter-faqs-12-10-2012.pdf.
22. Estimates for the insurance coverage provisions of the affordable care act updated for the recent supreme court decision. July 2012. http://www.cbo.gov/sites/default/files/cbofiles/attachments/43472-07-24-2012-CoverageEstimates.pdf.
23. Kaiser Commission on Medicaid and the Uninsured. Medicaid eligibility, enrollment simplification, and coordination under the affordable care act: a summary of CMS' March 23, 2012 final rule. Henry J. Kaiser Family Foundation. December 2012. http://www.kff.org/medicaid/upload/8391.pdf.
24. Olson LK. The politics of Medicaid. New York, NY: Columbia University Press; 2010.

Chapter 16
Next Experiments in ACA Legislation and Policy

John McDonough

In politics, it is much easier to play defense than offense. Those trying to enact major legislation in the face of fierce opposition must win every test and every battle. The opposition only has to win once to send everything crashing down to the point where you have to start all over again.

So it is with the struggle for healthcare reform in the USA. The Affordable Care Act (ACA) had to make its way through five standing committees in the US Congress despite fierce resistance at every stage: the Ways and Means, Energy and Commerce, and Education and Labor Committees in the US House, and the Finance Committee and the Health, Education, Labor, and Pensions Committees in the US Senate. After initial passage, the outcomes in both chambers then had to be reconciled. The ACA could have died in any one of these phases, and did not. But even after the ACA was duly passed and signed into law, it remains vulnerable to being overturned or undermined in a variety of ways.

An early and compelling post-enactment obstacle to the ACA came in the form of the constitutional challenges on which the Supreme Court ruled on June 28, 2012, upholding the law's individual mandate and its care and payment delivery reforms though overturning its mandatory state expansion of Medicaid. In the aftermath of the Supreme Court decision, the 2012 congressional and presidential elections became a kind of referendum on the ACA, unlike any in American legislative history, with Republicans vowing to repeal it if voters gave them the chance to do so.

Regardless of what happened in the elections, the end of 2012 brought the prospect of other major setbacks as the President and Congress wrestled with the federal fiscal challenges involving mandatory budget reductions through the sequestration process enacted in August 2011, the expiration of the 2001 and 2003 tax cuts, the continuing challenges with Medicare physician payment cuts, and more.

J. McDonough, D.P.H., M.P.A. (✉)
Center for Public Health Leadership, Harvard School of Public Health, Boston, MA, USA
e-mail: Jmcdonough@hsph.harvard.edu

H.P. Selker and J.S. Wasser (eds.), *The Affordable Care Act as a National Experiment:*   143
Health Policy Innovations and Lessons, DOI 10.1007/978-1-4614-8351-9_16,
© Springer Science+Business Media New York 2014

The story of the US health system and its continuing pursuit of equity and efficiency doesn't end there, no matter what the President, Congress, the courts, or states choose to do in late 2012 and early 2013 about the ACA and the federal budget. The ACA is one element of the broad agenda to make American healthcare equal to that in the rest of the developed world in fairness, efficiency, outcomes, and population health. Those of us who favor reform need to recognize that the reform struggle will play out over the next decade, and longer, whether the short-term outlook for the ACA in 2012–2013 is win, lose, or draw.

I like to consider health reform in stages. The stages are not sequential in a hard and fast way. And though the stages inevitably overlap, they help us to envision the components of comprehensive health reform and how we can achieve them. As I see them, the stages of healthcare reform are:

- Health reform 1.0 — Access: coverage, affordable and quality health insurance, service availability
- Health reform 2.0 — Delivery system reform: quality, efficiency, value, safety, workforce, health information technology
- Health reform 3.0 — Prevention: wellness, public/population health
- Health reform 4.0 — Health in all policies

Various titles within the ACA involve all four of these stages. So do health reform efforts in states such as Massachusetts and Vermont.

Starting with health reform 1.0, access, it is frequently asserted that coverage does not equal access, implying that those who struggle to achieve whatever form of universal health insurance are missing the point. While it is true that insurance coverage does not always guarantee access, it is foolhardy to suggest that coverage is unnecessary to enable real access. In the US context, it is impossible to have full and genuine access without coverage in some way.

Of the 25 most advanced nations, everyone except the USA has long demonstrated that it is possible to achieve universal healthcare coverage in a fiscally sustainable way. For a long time now, no other advanced country on the planet has allowed its citizens and residents to suffer financial ruin because they get sick. Yet that is still commonplace in the US. My home state of Massachusetts is the first to demonstrate that near-universal coverage is in fact achievable in the US context.

Some claim that Massachusetts will always be a healthcare policy outlier. After near-universal coverage became law in Massachusetts in 2006, I sometimes joked that we had taken a chain saw to the state and chopped around the border — and then we began floating toward Switzerland — because right now we look a lot more like Switzerland than any other place in the USA as far as healthcare is concerned.

The ACA faces severe implementation challenges simply because of the size and complexity of the American healthcare system. Beyond that is cultural resistance in the form of libertarian opposition to mandates. There is ongoing political resistance to the financing of reform, something I believe significantly underexplored as an explanation why health reform has been so hard to achieve in the USA as wealthier Americans begin facing major new tax increases in 2013 to pay for the ACA. And then there are enormous policy challenges owing to the variation across states.

One key challenge to long-term comprehensive health reform will be the residual uninsured. Assuming the ACA is implemented as well as the Congressional Budget Office (CBO) thought possible in the summer of 2012, we will still have 24 million uninsured Americans in 2019. There will not yet be universal coverage across the nation as there now is in Massachusetts.

Regarding access and coverage, we now face a new cost sharing reality. Democrats often say that Republicans lack a vision for health reform. I think they do have a vision and I believe they are advancing toward achieving that vision.

The Republican vision of health reform is simple: health insurance should be like auto insurance. That is, it should only pay for serious, severe, catastrophic incidents when patients suffer significant hard and high costs. The rest of the time, the cost of care should be out of pocket, on your own dime, with insurance covering nothing.

One of the most important developments in US healthcare over the past five–10 years has been the dramatic growth in levels of cost sharing for people with insurance. The rise in cost sharing helps generate the huge crowds at free rural healthcare clinics, where people line up for hours for treatment offered by volunteer physicians, dentists, and nurses. Surveys show that as many as 40 % of those visiting these clinics have health insurance. Their deductibles and coinsurance requirements are so high, however, it's not affordable for them to visit a medical professional in the normal course of events. So they stand in line with uninsured folks at free clinics for care often offered in barn stalls. This is a reality of healthcare in America today. And it will be even more a reality tomorrow as the crisis of the underinsured supplants the crisis of the insured.

More and more Americans are living with health insurance policies that expose them to significant financial risk. The ACA will ameliorate some of this trend, and some of the risk will continue to grow. Those who do not qualify for free or subsidized health insurance coverage under the ACA will continue to see increases in their deductibles and co-payments. And because of changes made to the final version of the ACA in 2010 to bring it within congressionally mandated spending limits, cost sharing for those eligible for insurance subsidies under the law will increase dramatically beginning in 2020. Thus even if the ACA overcomes the obstacles facing it in 2012 and 2013, there will still be serious affordability challenges for tens of millions who have health insurance.

If Republicans were successful in the November 2012 elections so that they could repeal the ACA in 2013, what would happen to health reform 1.0 and its improvements in coverage and access? Would there be a basis for Republican–Democratic compromise on new health reform?

To answer that question we must remember that in opposing the ACA, Republicans repudiated their own brain child, most notably a 180° turnaround on the individual mandate. Though it was a Republican think tank, the Heritage Foundation, that first proposed an individual mandate in 1989, an editorial in the *Wall Street Journal* on June 15, 2012, purported to explain "why the Democrats cooked up the individual mandate in the first place." Republicans are making a concerted attempt to erase the true history of the individual mandate.

So when Republicans advance ideas to reform healthcare, whether it's the Ryan plan rolling back Medicare entitlements or altering the deductibility of employer-based health insurance, we must be cautious before engaging in deals. Because down the line, they may repeat what they did in the summer of 2009—a 180° turn abandoning their own proposals rather than allow Democrats any success, bipartisan or otherwise, in health reform.

One thing that can't be an option is walking away from health reform. There is no walking away. If Republicans succeed in repealing the ACA, they will own every bad thing that happens in American healthcare for a long time to come. And the end result could still be positive health system reform, but only if we have the courage to stay with our convictions.

Turning to health reform 2.0, delivery system reform, it is well documented that among advanced nations, the US spends the most and gets the least value in quality and efficiency. One thing we are somewhat good at is using data and recognizing our flaws. In May, I presented to a group of Latin American health system leaders and spent the first 20 minutes showing some horrible data about US health system performance. Several audience members remarked to me at the conclusion that they could never speak about the flaws of their own systems in such a public way.

It is perhaps our saving grace that we are willing to talk about what a mediocre, flawed, inefficient, and poor value healthcare system we have in the USA. That gives us a basis for system reform. One thing that Massachusetts reform shows is that the passage of near-universal coverage in 2006 did not lead people into a rabbit hole pretending that the system problems did not matter anymore. If anything, Massachusetts' reform triggered an urgent, realistic, and pragmatic conversation about cost containment. The result is that, as of 2012, the Massachusetts Legislature now has passed three cost containment laws following onto the 2006 law. We are the first state in the nation looking at macro spending limits on medical care, something never contemplated meaningfully in any other state or the federal government.

Massachusetts' three cost containment laws, like Title III of the ACA, generate experiments to explore ways to deliver high-quality care at lower cost or at least to lower cost growth trends. The ACA also sets a powerful agenda for long-term reform with the system improvements embedded in Title III.

Two Title III reforms that I find provocative are, first, the penalties on hospitals for readmissions within 30 days and, second, the penalties on hospitals with high rates of hospital-acquired infections. I see these as part of a family of delivery system reforms that begin to move us beyond pay for performance and toward paying for outcomes. Readmissions and hospital-acquired infections are just the start. There is a range of potentially preventable events: readmissions, admissions, emergency department visits, complications during an inpatient stay, and outpatient procedures. These are all delivery system categories for which we have data systems and structures in place now to enable us to incentivize providers based on outcomes rather than fee-for-service volume. How this will be done is still uncertain, but we are definitely starting down this road.

Health reform 3.0 is prevention, wellness, and public health. We know, fundamentally, that healthcare costs rise not so much because of our healthcare delivery system. They are rising, most of all, because of the explosion of chronic disease. And we know that most chronic disease is tied to people's behaviors, particularly diet and nutrition, exercise, substance abuse, and other related activities. Right now about 11 % of all American adults have type 2 diabetes. The trend suggests that by 2020, the rate will be about 20 %. These estimates are staggering figures for a disease with potentially life-threatening consequences that is preventable and reversible.

The problem is not just diabetes. It is the burden of illness in those with multiple chronic diseases. We can devote immense resources to improving quality and efficiency in the care delivery system. Yet if we don't address prevention, wellness, and population health challenges, we will not win.

Title IV of the ACA contains the beginnings of a national attempt to improve prevention and wellness through such measures as the creation of the Public Health and Prevention Trust, a national prevention strategy, and calorie labeling on menus. We can see similar measures emerging in the healthcare reform dialogue in Massachusetts.

To date we have not seen real political mobilization around these prevention and wellness efforts. We have not yet seen real public pressure at either the federal or state levels to create a meaningful prevention agenda. But the potential for such pressure is building. One example is the food movement in Brooklyn, New York (Brooklyn would be the third largest city in the USA if it were its own municipality). In 2008, the Brooklyn Food Coalition held its first summit/conference, a daylong series of teach-ins and other activities around nutrition and healthy eating with more than 3,000 attendees. At their recent event in spring 2012, they had 5,000 attendees.

There is power in this emerging food movement. We haven't yet figured out how to channel it effectively into a political mobilization to overcome the entrenched power of the agribusiness and food industries, which will do whatever they can to prevent us from influencing people to eat in healthier ways. But we can hope for positive change as the food movement matures and develops popular support.

The final stage of reform, health reform 4.0, is also exemplified in the ACA and takes prevention, public health, and wellness to the next level by adopting the "health in all policies" approach. The impetus for this has been growing for more than a decade, and we've already seen some states move in this direction.

In January 2009, Massachusetts launched a health-in-all-policies program called Mass in Motion, run by the state's Department of Public Health. Its goal is to promote healthy diet and exercise habits by combining resources across state government. Another example is California, where in February 2010 then-Governor Arnold Schwarzenegger signed an executive order calling for a health-in-all-policies approach. But we need to take health-in-all-policies to another level.

The ACA's Title IV, which addresses prevention and public health, requires the creation of an annual national prevention strategy. The first version was released in June 2011, and it is an amazing document, not just in what it says but in how it was drafted.

Surgeon General Regina Benjamin chaired the group that created the document, and sitting around her table were representatives from the department of health and human services, as one might expect. Also sitting at that table were officials from the departments of agriculture, defense, education, housing and urban development, homeland security, interior, justice, labor, transportation, and veterans affairs, as well as other federal agencies and offices. It was the first real effort in the nation's history to establish a population health agenda that involves the span of federal governmental functions. It reflects an understanding that if we don't deal with transportation issues, for example, we will never improve health as we want.

The Massachusetts consumer advocacy group, Healthcare For All, was instrumental in getting Massachusetts state legislators to form any state's first-ever prevention caucus. About 50 legislators meet regularly to discuss prevention issues, and they are looking at how to take the national prevention strategy and translate it into a Massachusetts prevention strategy. When we think about healthcare reform, we think about insurance coverage, delivery system and payment reforms, and public health. The gold standard for healthcare reform should be health-in-all-policies.

Regardless of what happens in the short term between 2012 and 2013, whether the news for healthcare reform is good or bad, whether we're scratching our heads to try to figure out if it's good or bad, one way or another we have lots of work ahead of us. With that in mind I will close by sharing a lesson I learned from Don Berwick in 1991, when he was co-leading the National Demonstration Project on Quality Improvement in Healthcare, yet to become the Institute for Healthcare Improvement. He taught me, "every defect is a treasure." That is because every defect presents the opportunity to improve things and make things better. If you can't learn to recognize the defects, how will you ever improve anything?

We see so many defects in our health system. Yet they all point to where we need to go next and ways to get there. Whatever happens next, let's keep moving.

Chapter 17
Epilogue

Harry P. Selker

As outlined in this volume, the ACA is itself an experiment on a massive scale, and it also supports explicit healthcare delivery and policy research. Both are important. It is true that "something had to be done" to improve access to healthcare in this country, so the experimental intervention was put in place, and we as a society will evaluate it (along with the Office of the Assistant Secretary of Health and Human Services (HHS) for Evaluation and others). Continued improvements will benefit from the experiments with rapid-cycle evaluation supported by the Centers for Medicare and Medicaid Services (CMS) Innovation Center and by research on treatments and care strategies supported by Patient Centered Outcomes Institute (PCORI). All available information will be important in adjusting and optimizing the ACA's initial approaches.

The implementation of the changes by the ACA is vast. As reviewed in Shawn Bishop's chapter, the ACA has effects across the healthcare system. In healthcare insurance, it substantially expands coverage, provides financial subsidies for individuals and small employers, and creates insurance market exchanges, and at CMS it reduces the growth rate in Medicare payment rates for most services and creates new incentives and requirements in the payment for care in Medicare and Medicaid. Also, it expands significantly the ability to eliminate fraud and abuse in Medicare/Medicaid. It has aspects that raise funds for special purposes, such as taxes on medical manufacturers and insurers that support PCORI, and increased Medicare taxes on individuals with higher income. In influencing direct care, it has measures to enhance the safety of care delivered in the system and aims to achieve cost savings through improvements in care rather than only by price reductions, even while moving the US healthcare system away from a fee-for-service model. Aiming at

H.P. Selker, MD, MSPH (✉)
Tufts Clinical and Translational Science Institute, Tufts University, Boston, MA, USA

Institute for Clinical Research and Health Policy Studies, Tufts Medical Center,
Boston, MA, USA
e-mail: hselker@tuftsmedicalcenter.org

H.P. Selker and J.S. Wasser (eds.), *The Affordable Care Act as a National Experiment:*   149
Health Policy Innovations and Lessons, DOI 10.1007/978-1-4614-8351-9_17,
© Springer Science+Business Media New York 2014

the public's health over the long term, it has an increased emphasis on disease detection and prevention and has new authority and funds for public health programs. In rebalancing the US healthcare workforce, it grows education and training support for healthcare providers in critical areas, including primary care. And it directly touches the US healthcare system in many other ways as well. Finally, the ACA has created research entities, the CMS Innovation Center and PCORI, to inform and improve implementation of the ACA and the entire healthcare system.

This vast experiment is just getting under way, and yet already its consequences on the healthcare system, writ large, and on the national political dialogue the have been profound. The impact in neither realm is close to complete. One hopes that these transformations will enhance and sustain the effectiveness and vitality of the US healthcare system; however the results are only just beginning to be evident. The passage of the ACA was just the beginning of the experiment of transforming American healthcare—and there is far more left to do and learn.

Index